One Gift of Grace

ISBN: 1-4196-4769-5
Library of Congress Control Number: 2006905426

To order additional copies, please contact us.
BookSurge, LLC
www.booksurge.com
1-866-308-6235
orders@booksurge.com

DR. J.R. SMITH

ONE GIFT OF GRACE

My Path Through to the Other Side of Disease

2006

One Gift of Grace

TABLE OF CONTENTS

ACKNOWLEDGEMENTS

No one finishes a story, or even begins a story without many souls around. I have no way to tell each and every person that entered my life journey thank you. Take this as my attempt to name a few and I hope the rest know what they have meant by my acknowledgement somewhere along the path.

Firstly and lastly I thank God for carrying me through from the beginning of this journey until today.

At the beginning, middle and present my family, each and everyone, from parents to siblings to nieces and nephews, to cousins; they know how deeply I love them all. My father, though gone from us, is still with me and I could not have finished the journey I started without the strength his life force instilled in me and my siblings.

To the doctors and medical staff of Vanderbilt University Hospital Stem Cell Transplant Unit, Dr. Chapman's surgical group, and the Pulmonologists and their surgical group, your knowledge and your skills have made my continued existence richer and obviously more permanent. Thank you for tolerating me at my worst and healing my broken body. Your life gifts of strong intellect and your desire to solve difficult problems and your conviction to your practice is remarkable. I was blessed to be in your care.

To my friends, your support during the good and bad let me know I was and continue to be valued in this life.

To Mark for continuing to be a friend and for all the support before and after the fact.

To the staff at the in-between clinic, you gave me space to approach my future and a place to be occupied with things other than myself.

To Sharon and Melissa, thanks for getting me back onto a horse.

To the staff and doctors at Animal Medical and Laser Surgical Center for taking a chance on a recovering vet. Your grace around your welcoming me into your fold has touched my heart.

To doctors Rhea Morgan and Tracey King for taking such wonderful care of Topper at a time I was pretty helpless.

To Susan and David Porterfield, two wonderfully generous and loving people with whom I have been blessed to call friend.

To Avi Askey, friend and the creator of my little Garden of Eden, a joy I can experience every day.

To Anne Powers for teaching me to just let go, see the different view and let the paint flow!

To Allison Brown at BookSurge for helping me to find the way into print: your persistence kept me moving toward the final form.

To Jim Knox for your professional critique and encouraging words, and Dr. Madan Jagasia for your medical correctness proofing: thanks for the help along the way toward the final form of this story.

Thanks to my sister Rebecca, who tried to read it but could only cry. That emotion helped me realize I had brought truth to the work.

I thank the good people of Rockwood United Methodist Church, the churches of my friends and family, for the prayers and the support they lent me and my family during and after this trial.

To the poetry of Mattie Stepanek, his grace and insight gave me courage.

God Bless you all, I will never be the same because of your influence on my life. Thank you.

I Dedicate This Book To Two Very Important Groups In My Life.

To My Foils:
Myself, AMM, Transplant, Lung Disease And Dr. Aaron Milstone
And

To My Heroes:
My Family, Dr. Madan Jagasia, And Dr. Aaron Milstone

FOREWORD

In January of 2000, an unexpected push deflected my step onto a different life path. The force of that push has not abated in intensity; it has changed focus from time to time and continues to bring trials and periods for self-discovery. Consequences along this path have been many but I have found the blessings received and gifts given and received much greater than any suffered consequence.

Consider this an invitation to share my travels through the last few years as I attempt a reconstruction of those days. Forgive my tendency to let my philosophy, though sometimes convoluted, prevail. The requirement of my reliving the past is to make sense of that past so to go on with my future. The hope is to help someone else, if even marginally, on a similar journey.

Do not think I hold my self either an expert or a great writer in any fashion. I am just a traveler and storyteller on this quest of sharing my lessons with those who want to know the story.

Some areas of the journey are spotty in my mind; so family members relived their perceptions of the passage for clarification. Some names and places have been changed, for I have no intention of representing anything except my reaction to my life as I perceived it in that moment of living. Some of those moments were harsh and eye-opening. I pray you find some truth for your life in this difficult journey. If not, I hope you enjoy the ride.

CHAPTER ONE

"This is who I am made of..."

Children can come at odd times and in strange places. My arrival was in a bleak province of a foreign country to two very American parents. The birth occurred in Newfoundland, Canada; the family: United States Air Force.

My father, Major Jack F. Smith, was an active duty USAF pilot for over 20 years. He served in the 416th Bomb Group of light bomber pilots, A-20's and A-26's, during the Second World War: Mace's Aces, I believe. He and my mother, Rosalie, married after the war, in 1950. The result of this marriage was five children: two boys (Jack, Larry), and three girls (Laura, Becky, and me). Larry and Laura are twins.

The decades of the '50s and '60s wove threads of their history into each of us children; as if stitching on the unattached quilt pieces that eventually would become our lives. Those years wove through our uncluttered existence and found us as children without care, slowly losing our innocence, finding our talents, understanding our future desires, always adventurous and staying mostly happy.

The decade of the '70s found us eager young adults unique in our politics, in our spirit, in our attitudes, in our lives and loves. This uniqueness in our life quilts does have one common woven thread: love. We love each other, warts and all.

As service brats, we grew toward each other. Moving every four years taught us that in the end our family was the comfort we would cling to through life. Friends, though wonderful and necessary people, come and go. Family is indispensable, and steadfastness to your roots a virtue.

My parents' families were firmly rooted in southern tradition and the Methodist faith. Dad was born and raised in the Winton Chapel community of the town of Rockwood, Tennessee. His father, E.D. "Dode" Smith, was a farmer who tended a large acreage of Tennessee River "bottom land." He was elected multiple times as justice of the peace, was on the county court for 30 years and was a state representative.

Dad's mother, Nell, was the city-raised daughter of one of Rockwood's pioneer families. My greatgrandfather, I.G. Fleming, was one of Rockwood's first dentists. Her mother, Ida B. Lasater Fleming, was the daughter of a Reconstruction-era state senator and early member of the city of Manchester, Tennessee. She was known for her intense support of the local Methodist church.

The Smith family was large, four boys (Dick, Jack, Bill, and Pat) and one girl (Willie Frances). They were boisterous, fun-loving pranksters, hardworking, intelligent and community servants all their lives. The boys served in WWII in the Army, Air Force and Navy. Dick, a submariner on the USS Corvina, did not come home. Aunt Frances (Cissy) helped in the defense industry in Baltimore, Maryland, building the planes her brothers flew. She returned home after Dick died and went to work for the postal service. Granddaddy died in January of 1945, three months before his other boys started to come home from the war.

My mother, Rosalie Graves, was the last child of 10 born to Benjamin Audley and Laura Emily. Her siblings were four boys (Benton, Audley, Dutch and Bill) and five girls (Kit,

Muriel, Verne, Henrietta, Frankie). She lived in Sale Creek, Tennessee.

Her mother's family was one of the first families in Hamilton County. Her father's family was a mix of native Hamilton County and Michigan. They were loving, hardworking sharecroppers, religious, funny, earnest, smart yet stoic people. Mom lived first as wife and mother and secondly as a nurse. She graduated about 1943 from the Baroness Erlanger School of Nursing in Chattanooga, Tennessee.

Our parents raised us to be mindful in our choices and to remember that each action has its consequence. Recognizing those consequences and understanding them, we lived with the result. Mom and Dad raised their children to be productive citizens and to find profitable ways of supporting themselves. They taught us work was genderless. Our parents raised children who came to believe as adults what they taught us: God and family, home and hard work first. We all went to college gladly, all of us have advanced degrees, and all of us have done well, however one defines well.

Life choices in the family lie in medicine and business. Jack is a partner in one of the nation's largest accounting firms. He is married and has two children. Larry is a medical doctor whose specialty is ENT surgery. He is married and the father of three. Laura chose to follow along our parents' life path. Laura is both a Major in the United States Air Force and a nurse. She married and, fortunately for me, had no children. My youngest sister, Becky, is a senior vice president at a national investment management company. She is not married, and that leaves me.

CHAPTER TWO

"My life in a nutshell"

Nineteen-fifty-three brought a new child into the Smith household, a child who was born loving horses, was athletic, hated to fly, was loving in nature, forthright, very curious, very sensitive to the comments and actions of others, and eager to please.

This child rode three or four rocking horses till their springs popped off the frame. She used at least a million pieces of colored chalk decorating the sidewalk leading to the front door with pictures of horses. The obsession with this beast left her pestering her father for a horse of her own, not knowing that the request was impossible to fill. With the military lifestyle, we moved every three or four years. That child didn't understand the concept of restraint and each lovingly offered "not now, baby" stung her heart and made the dream that much more desirable.

That child became me. Not much has changed, really. I still love the magnificence of horses, am still curious, still caring and still sensitive, frank to a fault, and sometimes, well, oftentimes, downright clueless. The difference is that the focus of that childlike sensitivity has shifted over time from my physical self to my spirit, life issues, my family, my friends and my passions of learning to paint, writing, riding horses and practicing veterinary medicine.

My first incarnation was as a research chemist. In 1975, I

graduated from Tennessee Technological University with a B.S. in Chemistry. My first job took me into the world of pesticide manufacturing, an environment of exposure to chemicals such as benzene, toluene, organophosphates, chlorine and multiple other compounds. Environmental conditions at this facility were so corrosive the cars would lose their paint. Two years of living in this poor air quality made going back for an advanced degree in Organic Chemistry seem appropriate and, frankly, I felt, life-saving. I had had to escape one too many plumes of accidentally released chlorine gas and possible accidental poisoning with an organophosphate pesticide or asphyxiation by hydrogen sulfide gas. That life choice just did not fit, on many levels. The time to move on to the next stage of my life had arrived.

Dr. Eugene Kline at Tennessee Tech and research grants from Grand Forks North Dakota Energy Division sponsored the work that brought me back to Tech. My thesis dealt with one of the problems the center had recognized during the liquefaction of lignite coal.

This time around, polynuclear aromatic hydrocarbons were my poison of choice. The synthesis medium was dimethyl sulfoxide (DMSO). The skin easily absorbs whatever chemical is dissolved in DMSO.

Class work and research were finished in 1980. I went to work as a product development chemist, working with plasticizers and polymers and inks. The thesis was finished during the evenings after work and graduation was in 1982. I bought my horse during this time period; a stubborn, beautiful gray quarter horse.

After my degree was conferred, I started working in the energy field, a choice of specialty that left me at the mercy of the price of a barrel of oil. When oil was up, I had a research job. When oil prices were down, the lack of research funding in new energy futures made it difficult to find a job directly linked to new fuels research. The early '80s found me as a lab manager and troubleshooter in a pilot plant, developing a production protocol for coal slurry. The price of oil was up. The slurry was to be a substitute for a #6 fuel oil. After a year, the price of oil dropped, and the pilot plant was shut down.

The mid-'80s were spent on air cleaning methods, and using coal for dual level energy production at the University of Tennessee Space Institute. That research budget was tenuous at best.

By the fall of 1987, I began to realize I was not enjoying my career as a chemist. I had moved into lower management, writing research proposals and reports and had completely left basic research and bench work. I had always loved theoretical chemistry. Now my job was to see that others did the work. Even though successful in completing the projects, I found no joy here, and began to feel like a fraud. Another bad fit in the career department, but much personal growth had occurred.

Need I say more about my history of chemical exposure? I had always kept a professional approach, using gloves, masks, employing hoods and using common sense. Experience and education demanded that the chemicals worked with during those years be respected. Now was the time to let that world go for one that brought more satisfaction.

My love of animals, my curious nature and my interest in medicine began driving me in a different direction. While working at the institute I applied to and was accepted into the Veterinary College at the University of Tennessee. This was 1988. I reluctantly sold my horse.

CHAPTER THREE

"Oh, yeah, I already told you that horses are my weak spot."

In August of 1988 I entered vet school bright-eyed and full of anticipation. Having been out of the classroom since 1980, many behavioral adjustments had to be made to ramp up my study ethic. Classes were credited at 21-24 hours a semester and information was doled out at an accelerated pace. Veterinarians treat a lot of species, all with somewhat different anatomy, and not all of them react the same way to similar situations or respond to the same medications. Much had to be learned in a short time. The students in my class all worked hard, played hard and spent many hours together building our knowledge and our skills.

The first two summer semesters were free time for underclass students. The summer of 1989 I worked at UTCVM for a veterinary pathologist, trying to separate bovine growth factors.

My second summer, in 1990, I did not work. Realizing the next two years would be very demanding, I wanted one last summer before the onslaught. Relaxation and spending time with my family were the priorities. As always, the Smith farm would be a scene of much of this relaxation.

The Smith farm is located on Watts Bar Lake. TVA was born in the '40s and the dam system left the majority of land in that region underwater, including my father's childhood home. Cissy, my dad's sister, and Uncle Bill, my dad's brother, lived on the piece that had not been covered up during the dam and river formations. We lived in town in the Fleming home. Childhood summers were spent on that farm. And as children, we loved nothing more than staying the night with our Aunt Cissy. Life around her was always an adventure.

Cissy lived in the old cabin that the Smith family had built in the 1940s. She had added on to the cabin with time, but as children, we still used the outhouse. We formed the "pee-can potty patrol" every morning and our "responsibility" was to empty the thunder-pots from the night before.

The outhouse, a single-holer, was housed in a wooden shed lined with tar paper. It stood at the end of a gravel path about 100 feet from the house. The forced march to go potty could stand your hair on end, especially if the lights along the path were out. Winter cold nipping at your backside certainly encouraged one to finish in a hurry.

Summer was creepy. Being children of the South, we had a tendency to want to tell tall tales, make the grown-ups laugh and our siblings and cousins jealous; the johnnie excursion was certainly fodder. A simple visit instantly became a terrible life-threatening experience, fueled with visions of big hairy spiders, "waspers," stinky ol'skunks and huge poisonous snakes lurking along the knee-high grassy path and dangling in the darkened corners of the johnnie house. Never mind the errant sibling or cousin lurking in wait for the next visitor. All of the Smith cousins became great pranksters, good sprinters and probably exaggerators as a result. Never a day or night went by without an episode of near-death.

"Run! There is something in there!"

One forlorn cry of a cousin or sibling would set us to the

path away from the john if heading there, or to it, to see what was happening, or from behind it doubled over in hysterics. Sometimes, our legs could not carry us fast enough. The gravel set on the path became huge boulders or thick slime, causing us to struggle and slip as we ran toward safety. Cis would stand at the screen door encouraging us while laughing and waving us to the finish line. Her living room was our safe haven once again. Well, at least until the next morning, or maybe even that night!

Growing up, the Smith cousins spent many hours playing, hiking, swimming, skiing, learning to drive, farming, baling and stacking hay, picnicking and just being kids at this farm. Cissy taught all the cousins about the trees and flowers and snakes and bugs, and how to build a good fire, how to work smart and hard and to have fun in the forest. Glad I was able to have the experiences growing up on that farm provided.

We always came back as we got older, and this summer was no different. Since I had sold my own horse before I went to vet school, I was searching for one to ride. Maybe Chris would let me ride her little mare.

Chris was Uncle Bill's adopted daughter, from his marriage to Judy after Aunt Gwen died. Chris had a young quarter horse named Pickpocket. She was a pretty little buck-skinned colored mare. One day while I was visiting Cissy, Chris mentioned her little mare.

"I don't ride her. Momma sent her to Spring City to be trained but she still is a handful."

Must be fate; I was holding my breath, hoping she said yes to my next question, oblivious to anything but the bliss of riding a horse.

"Well, I have some time this summer. Do you want me to try to ride her?"

"Sure, if you want to, I don't care. Any time, you just have to catch her."

"Thanks, Chris."

Giggling inside, I started the climb up the hill to Cissy's house. I turned around and looked out to the right, trying to make a decision. Below the cabin was the barn, and to the right of the barn a nice flat hay field. I chose this field as my riding area. I stepped up on to the screened-in porch.

"Hey, Cis!"

"Youuuuh!" Cissy was in the older part of the cabin. But even so her voice shattered the silence in response. She sounded like a dinner bell peeling across the fields, a sound I had grown up to respond to and respect. When one of the elder Smiths gave out a holler, you really could hear it all over the farm. The lake would then echo those calls and magnify them so that as children we never could get out of earshot, even if we tried, and we did try.

"Do you have some stakes and some old plastic plates?"

"Sure, why? What you gonna' do, girlie?"

"Well, I thought I'd stake out an area so I could ride Pickpocket for Chris."

"Hey, yeah, let's do it!"

Cissy busied herself in the cabinets and found all the plates and stakes and string we would need. We grabbed a couple of hammers and headed out the door. Cissy always had whatever you could possibly think of.

"Let's go!"

Off we went down the hill to the hay field. I am sure we looked like Mutt and Jeff. I am 5'10" tall while Cis was only about 5'3". We measured off the arena by our foot length, placed the stakes, roped off, plated and labeled them with letters like a dressage arena would have. We walked over the area, made sure there were no holes to step in, and called it done.

"Great, I'll see ya tomorrow, thanks for helping Cis."

That next afternoon I was ready. I put on my breeches and my tall boots. Grabbed my saddle, girth, pad and bridle and put it in the car. The family had gathered to celebrate the 4th of July. Mom, Becky, Larry, Daddy and I drove down to Cissy's. Mom and Cis and Becky visited, Daddy worked on his tractor. Larry helped Dad on the tractor, but that did not last long. Being a surgeon, Larry was not very eager to be using wrenches and pulling out bolts that did not want to budge. His hands were his life; he had to take care of them and tractors were known knuckle busters. Uncle Bill was working in the barn. Chris was not home.

I saddled Pickpocket and led her out to the field. The day was already July hot and the lake's nearness made it so humid that every creature around was slick with moisture. Almost as if that river was intentionally reaching up out of its banks with liquid tendrils to grab onto our skin and ooze into our pores, engulfing every object in its way.

I put the long line on Pick and trotted her out. "Handful" was an apt definition, as she was already bucking and snorting while under the saddle. The next circle on the line, every dog on the property was coming in to bark and chase the horse's heels. Pickpocket began bowing up, snorting and flaring her nostrils, breathing hard and glaring all wide-eyed. Darn dogs. Cissy, Becky and Uncle Bill quickly arrived and removed those silly dogs.

Reaching the riding area the mare had calmed enough to ride. I rode through her gaits for about 45 minutes. She had done well, had responded nicely, and overall had behaved herself; a thoroughly enjoyed effort. We were both tired from the effort and Pickpocket was snorting with each step. She was quite relaxed while walking along the circle as we both cooled off from the exercise. An approaching voice amplified across the field.

"Hey! Janet. How'd she do?"

Chris was home. She was riding the old mare, we called her 42.

"She did real well."

Chris rode 42 into the area and got in line behind me and Pickpocket. A feeling of unease swept over me.

"Chris, don't let 42 run up behind Pick. She isn't used to carrying someone on her back yet."

"Okay."

Still being a kid, Chris had the reputation of not listening very well sometimes. I looked over my shoulder and Chris and 42 were less than three feet behind Pickpocket's heels.

42 stuck her neck out, squealed and nipped Pickpocket's haunches. Pickpocket screamed back and, bowing up into a ball with all four feet off the ground, she kicked out behind and made contact with the older mare's chest. 42 screamed back and I felt another hard bump into Pick's rear.

The trees blurred as I felt hard ground on my knee, shoulder and wrist. Pickpocket was pinning my leg. My ankle found its way between the stirrup and the horse. My knee must have found a rock.

Stunned, I let go of the rein. Pick immediately gathered herself, rolled onto her chest, and stood up. Luckily, my foot was not caught in the stirrup. Shaking off the fall Pickpocket just stood there, turning her head in my direction, looking down at the idiot that was once on her back.

The fog of the fall lifted as Chris's scream brought me back to reality and found me relieved that Pickpocket hadn't decided to bolt right over me.

"Janet, Are you OK? Daaaddy! Daddy!"

As she was screaming, Cissy, Becky, Mom and Larry were running down the hill. Uncle Bill was coming across from the barn.

"Yeah, but it hurts. Is Pick Ok? How about you? 42?"

"Just fine."

Managing to pry myself off the ground, regaining my bearings and balance, I looked Pickpocket over for cuts, bruises and lameness. She was fine, a small bruise on her side where the stirrup had caught between her and the ground, but fine. I noticed Dad had left his tractor work and walked the 50 feet to the place of the fall.

Dad was a tall man about 6'3", thin, shiny white hair, big blue eyes, strong hands, broad shoulders, and he spoke with a deep, almost Scottish-accented voice that oozed Southern calmness and strength. He was a gentle loving soul, but could fight like a banshee for what he believed in. That was mostly his kids; seems we were his and Mom's life. He always wore overalls at the farm, and his worn, greasy, sweat-stained hat perched on his head. Dad heard the commotion and responded, always quietly in control, or so it seemed to me.

"Gal, you alright?"

"Yeah, Daddy, I'm fine but my knee really hurts, I feel a little shaky."

Tears were filling my eyes. I was responding to that voice. And even though I was 35, I reacted as Daddy's little girl. I was hurt. He had come, as so many times before, to fix the problem.

"Well, get that horse back to the barn and get your leg checked out."

"I will. I think I'll just go on home. Larry can look at it then. See ya later, Pa."

"Take your Momma with you."

"OK."

I limped toward the barn, the horse quietly in tow, snorting only occasionally with her body motion; Mom, Becky, Cissy and Larry saw I was standing and headed back up the hill. Uncle Bill was meandering in my direction from the barn. We met up about a third of the way back.

Uncle Bill, like Dad, had on his well-worn hat and a pair of old dungarees. He, like Cis, was short, about 5'8", with graying curly hair. An electrical engineer, he did not mince words often and had a great and very dry sense of humor. He began shaking his head before he reached me.

"Here, Janet, give me that damn horse. What are you trying to do, kill it?"

"Yeah, how'd you know?"

"This horse doesn't know how to work. It just stands around and eats all day and half the night. Boy, that sure was a hard way to dismount, gal. Try stirrups next time."

"Great advice, Uncle Bill. I'll do that next time."

He gave me a big hug.

"Are you really OK there, gal?"

"Well, sort of; my leg really hurts."

Uncle Bill then emphasized "that damn horse" with a tobacco spit and took the reins from my hands. He led the way; I painfully limped behind, fighting off tears with every step. We took off the tack. Chris rode 42 back to the barn and let the horses out to graze, obviously none the worse for wear.

Hobbling up the hill to Cissy's, I put my tack in the trunk, grabbed my dog, got in my car and had Becky drive me home. Mom came with us. Driving away from the farm I mournfully looked at my "ring" one more time, knowing I would not be using it again.

CHAPTER FOUR

"The truth is in the consequence."

The evening was coming fast and I hobbled into the house and fell onto the couch.

"Janet, let's get those breeches off so we can look at your knee."

Becky grabbed my boot heels and pulled my tall boots to the floor. Mom grabbed the breeches legs and peeled them off like a corn shuck. The pain that came with the pressure release was almost enough to make me pass out.

"Ouch, Mom, it hurts!"

"Oh, Janet, this leg is swelling so fast; good thing you had those breeches on for a while. They may have really helped keep this damage down. I don't know, I wish Larry and Jack would come on."

My leg began shaking uncontrollably. Becky walked away, afraid she would pass out.

"I guess they did help, but I'm paying for it now. I need something. I'm gonna take an Excedrin or something. No tellin' what time Larry and Daddy will get home."

I put some shorts on and lay down on the couch with a blanket.

Larry and Daddy finally came in about dark and soon Larry was looming over me with his 6'4" frame. All he needed was one look at my self-inflicted misfortune and he immediately entered into his doctor "mode."

"Janet, let me look at it. I need to see if you have bled into the muscle."

I jerked back. Larry's hands were on my knee and the pain was intolerable as he pushed and prodded around the joint and stabbed his fingers into the muscle. My knee, twice its normal size, was red, purple, and hot and screamed of pain.

"No! Larry, don't! It hurts too much."

I pushed myself deeper into the couch, trying to get away from the tender, yet prying hands. Tears of pain and fear were running down my cheeks. On top of this, I was sensing Larry's patience with my lack of participation was wearing thin.

"Fine." Larry quit the prodding and looked at me with more than agitation.

"Janet, this can get serious. What have you got in the house for pain? It's a holiday. I cannot get you anything tonight. Maybe we should just go to the hospital."

"No, I'm OK, I took an Excedrin."

"What! Boy, Janet, that was smart!" He was laughing at me by now. "You know better than that."

I did, but I was not thinking too clearly at the time, so I goofed and added insult to injury.

"All I have is left-over Mepergan from my dental surgery."

"Where are they?" he said, shaking his head as he walked past me around the corner.

"In the medicine cabinet. I hate Mepergan, Larry. It really leaves me in a fog." He started a deep, mocking laugh, the kind that little brothers have when they finally get one up on you.

"You may be glad you are! Here, take two, no sense in you hurting, I don't let my patients hurt."

He handed me the burgundy-colored pills and a glass of water; Nirvana in a pill, soma for the masses. I obediently took the reality remover and handed the empty glass to Becky.

Larry had become the "Doctor" in a moment; he morphed back into my lil' brother with equal alacrity. This change meant the Smith behavior pattern of defining the litany of consequences, my lesson for the day, was beginning.

Becky was sitting nearby and was ready to add to the list if Larry just happened to forget a tasty morsel of knowledge. Mom and Dad said not a word.

Sitting at the foot of the couch, Larry touched my arm gently and changed his tone into that brotherly thing and sternly but compassionately began defining what I knew in my heart.

"You know, Janet, it is a good thing you are not in school right now. After this, you would not be able to walk, you would be on crutches. If you were in clinics, you would probably be kicked out of school because you couldn't function as a student has to on clinical rotation. You have chosen a new path. You can't do stupid things anymore. I know you love horses but you had better think twice from now on."

I should have paid attention to that red flag on the day Chris and I talked about Pickpocket. Larry was right. I had taken a risk because of my passion for horses. The consequences could be harsh. I made the choice to not ride again until after graduation.

The couch in the den was to become my new home; no way could I climb the stairs to my room. Mobility over the next few days was poor and I tended to stay on that couch too much. The posttrauma seroma was so large I could not flex my knee. Dr. Evans opened it and drained it. It began to heal and I could move a little easier.

One evening, about 10 days post-accident, I felt odd. My head ached and my skin burned. My feet finally found that unknown surface called the floor. I found a thermometer, and took my temperature, thinking my actions had gone unnoticed.

"I am going upstairs to take a cool bath." I hobbled out of the den heading upstairs to the big, deep, claw-foot bathtub.

Mom was sitting in her favorite chair, reading. Dad was in his chair, loudly watching TV. Before I got out the door the reaction came in a soft but determined tone.

"Why? What's your temperature?" The nurse was coming out of hiding.

"Oh, about 103.5."

Reacting to a Mother's demand I immediately wished I had not been so quick to answer.

"Well, I am calling Dr. Tom." Mom was on my heels as I headed off upstairs.

"Mom, you don't need to call him tonight. I'll be OK until the morning."

After sitting in the tub for about 10 minutes, Mom walked in with my orders from Dr. Evans.

"Go to the emergency room, they are expecting you."

I packed a few things and Dad drove me to the local hospital, about two blocks from the house.

That one blissful horse episode, followed by that one phone call of 15 minutes to my doctor, led to 10 days spent in the hospital battling pneumonia. Very ill, I slept most of the time.

During the course of the pneumonia, Dr. Evans treated me with IV antibiotics and respiratory therapy. Each passing day should have brought a decrease in my white count as the disease resolved. An odd thing I remember was that Dr. Evans kept commenting on how my white cell count did not seem to be dropping with therapy; it was hanging around 20-25,000. I lost 20 pounds, managed to be able to breathe again and was released from the hospital about a week before vet school classes started mid-August. It was a tough semester.

During my senior year, while on Large Animal Medicine clinic rotation, I was walking a mare and foal out to graze. My classmates were being goofy, laughing it up and trudging along behind the mare. There was a sense of calm by the time the mare got to the grass; I began to slowly let out the line so she could graze. The foal ran up behind its mom. Mom cut her eyes at me and in a nanosecond she cow-kicked and caught me on the inside of my leg. Larry's prediction had come true. I was on crutches for two weeks but I managed to get my work done and was not kicked out of school. You would think I would start to hate horses. I graduated in 1992.

CHAPTER FIVE

"Stop this world, let me off…"

Mose Allison

My first four years of veterinary practice found me in large clinics with six to 10 doctors, doing mixed animal work, with long hours, many cases and little sleep. The next six years were spent in smaller practices, doing small animal work with many cases and a little more sleep.

I went into this venture of practicing veterinary medicine already tired from four long years of pushing all the time. The next job would not change that situation. A busy practice in the Appalachians found me as the only doctor. One of the clients used to say upon his arrival, "1-800-Dr.-Janet."

I started working there in January 1996. The commute to work was an hour and a half, twice daily, 120 miles total, driving country roads. The nice thing about the drive was the view of Tennessee's valleys and mountains, a nice way to start and end a day. The bad part about the commute was getting behind slow tractors, winter cold, sudden ice storms and snow.

Once there, clients came every 15 to 20 minutes, and there were usually several surgeries daily. I enjoyed the job. I liked to be busy and felt I had developed a good bedside manner over the years of practice. My efficiency in gettting a job done was developed in industry and as result good diagnostic skills followed in kind. I had learned much during my first four years of practice, and this job showed me how much more I needed to learn. During the next six months, I adjusted to my busy lifestyle. Then the unthinkable happened.

In June 1996, six months after coming home, Dad suffered a massive coronary 10 days after his corneal transplant. He underwent bypass surgery but his heart was too weak and scarred to allow him to survive. He was in and out of consciousness throughout the ordeal so we were able to at least let him know how much we loved him and to say goodbye. Larry, Laura, Becky and I stood at Dad's beside while the nurse turned off his respirator and stopped the medicine that could not save his life. As his vital signs disintegrated from the screen, we said the 23rd Psalm and let him go.

That death was too hard for Mom to watch. Jack took her outside and away from her greatest moment of loss. When Dad was gone, Mom went back to his bedside so she could say her goodbyes in private. Mom and I drove home together.

My family was past damaged. The next two years were incredibly grief-filled for my mother and all of us children. Tears were always on the surface, each odor, a song, or piece of his clothing brought heart-wrenching sobs. Merely walking into his garage remains as difficult today as the day he died. Our rock is gone. Mr. Sunshine has died and now we have to reach deep and find him within us.

CHAPTER SIX

"The Awakening"

I continued to work in Appalachia for the next four years. One day near the end of 1999 there came a realization and an admission: I was awfully tired, angry, cranky, and insensitive to those around me. What was worse, I didn't care. I ached all over, my stomach was a mess, my feet were very painful, my legs were swelling and I was just past tired.

Was this grief from my Dad's death or burnout? I really wanted to get away from myself, and the job. There were days the staff wanted away from me as well. Who could blame them? I was probably a real pain to work with during that time.

Deanna, the clinic receptionist, was acting very distant with me one day. Deanna and I had become good acquaintances over those years. Not one to mince words, her actions became clear indicators of her mood. I liked that about Deanna. She was very surly that day, banging around, not speaking much. Something was on her mind, and that something seemed to be me.

While waiting for the next client, I was sitting at my desk and writing on charts. Deanna stomped into the treatment area, gave me a trite little message and started to turn and leave. Tired of the drama in the clinic life, the behavior all of us were suffering under at this time needed to end, the tension broken. An opportunity presented itself to end the whole charade. Why waste an opportunity?

"Deanna, do you have something to say to me? It isn't going to hurt my feelings, so let's have it."

She did. She, in just a few, angry choice words, told me her position about my attitude.

"You've changed!"

I looked her in the eye and smugly reacted to her comment.

"Do you feel better?"

"Yes, I do." Her face was red and her eyes wide. She left the treatment area still angry, but cooling down, heading back to her desk.

"Great, now let's all get back to work."

I heaved the proverbial internal sigh of relief. Everybody else seemed to be as a wild animal after being hit by receding headlights, wide-eyed, stunned and relieved the danger was gone.

I had changed; I was willing to own that behavior. My attitude was one driven by exhaustion, a desire to still do a good job and to be dependable. Tired beyond belief, I knew I had burned the candle at both ends for far too long and that behavior had set me up for a fall. Clients began to recognize the change in my demeanor and kept asking me not to leave the practice. I had made many nice acquaintances and loved caring for their pets, but I was so very tired, bone-tired.

Weighing too much, the summer through fall found me dieting and working out in the gym daily, grumbling and getting nowhere in my workout. I had lost 20 pounds but my abdomen was still very round. Eating ended in pain and serious heartburn. Small amounts of food created misery. A simple meal meant a painful hour of pacing, waiting for the stomach to empty. A warm shower ended with my body a mass of itching flesh. I was not hungry, had trouble sleeping and was too tired to enjoy life much anymore. Singing lessons were becoming very painful. One deep breath was difficult and it was hard to even take in enough air to hit a note. Something was going on, but what? Did I really, truly, want to know?

Around the beginning of January 2000, while trying to do the cardio parts of my exercise routine, my legs were like ton weights. My trainer really pushed me daily and today was no exception but I had had enough after only a few moments.

"John, I can't do this, I am just exhausted. My muscles will not go anymore."

John, a black belt in karate, did not have the phrase "give up" in his vocabulary. Today seemed different somehow.

"Well, let's try some lighter weights than what you have been doing. This is not like you to quit."

John handed me some 10-pound weights. After five reps, I was toast. I looked up at John and started shaking my head.

"Janet, let's call it a day; you might hurt yourself."

John's comment was reason enough to leave.

"I'll see you later."

The gym door closed behind and with my head hung low, realizing an element of fear not admitted before, I began to wonder what was coming this time. The workday finished, and we went home. What was wrong?

CHAPTER SEVEN

"Doctor, heal thyself! Trouble was I was a tired old horse doc."

Our family genetic history includes cardiovascular disease and cancer. Not just in my dad's family, but on both sides of the family. My first thought was heart problems. Dr. Evans did an EKG, found an arrythmia and referred me to a cardiologist at Baptist Hospital in Knoxville in January 2000. Dr. Bishop ordered the routine battery of tests: stress tests, ultrasound, radiographs, blood work, thallium scans, Holter monitor and uncertainty.

Two weeks later, the heart verdict came in. The clinic nurse showed me into an exam room, and pointed to a chair in front of an entire wall of glass. The view included the Tennessee River, UT's football stadium and parts of downtown Knoxville. Waiting for Dr. Bishop, I watched the cold February rain fall on the people walking outside. I was trying not to guess what was coming, and was emptying my head of those possibilities when the door opened.

Bishop was a tall, thin, dark-headed man: all business. He walked the short distance from the door to the desk and sat down. He adjusted the file and began looking at me over the top of his glasses.

"Janet, you need to see a hematologist, not me; your heart is basically sound. You do have a non-pathologic arrhythmia. We can try a beta-blocker and see if that helps slow it down and stop some of the VPCs. Your regular doctor can arrange a referral to a hematologist/oncologist."

Being a veterinarian, I found my doctors spoke to me without interpretation. I appreciated their respect for my knowledge base. I was someone who understood how their body was responding to its stresses. Respect has a doubled edge though, and sometimes I found that I wanted them to treat me as one who had no clue. As I was finishing this thought to myself, I saw Bishop was closing my file and pushing away from his desk.

Dr. Bishop stood up as casually as he came in, handed me a prescription for Propanolol, and walked out the door. Seems this quick session was over. I followed him out the door, he went straight; I turned left. He slowed and spoke over his shoulder.

"Call if you need anything. Hope all turns out well for you."

He was already halfway down the hall heading back into the clinic. Episode one, heart is fine, almost. A twinge of uncertainty and confusion welled deep in my chest.

"Thanks, doc. I appreciate your help."

Deep down though, all I thought was, well, that was informative!

I was still in the dark as to my exact medical state but a narrowing of information had begun. It was then that I sensed an understanding growing in my mind that the conversation with Dr. Bishop was the stick match starting the fuse for this new game. The match strike and that burning fuse left behind a lingering, sulfur-heavy, yellow-gray smoke that started hovering around my brain and left a noxious stinging odor in my nose. I didn't particularly care for that acrid smell. It reeked of the brimstone emanating from my unknown future hell.

I walked down the hall, head down, looking at the prescription Bishop had handed me so nonchalantly and plodded on to the patient checkout desk in a daze. What in the world was wrong?

It seemed my blood was creating a few problems. The "let's find the disease" game had begun and I found myself ultimately not so willing to play. Dr. Bishop referred me back to Dr. Evans to refer me to a hematologist/oncologist.

Being a procrastinator and one to rationalize, I put off the appointment. My elevated white count might be due to my infected hand, compliments of the latest dog bite I had received at work a few days before my stress test. I was on antibiotics and decided I would wait. This was February 2000. In the middle of March, I had a recheck visit with Dr. Evans at home. I was sitting on the exam table as usual when Dr. E walked in.

"Janet, I want you to go to the hem/onc department at Baptist. Your white count is still up and there are immature cells circulating."

He had that stern but concerned look on his face.

"Dr. Evans, I promise, when I get back from Toronto, I will go to see the oncologist."

I wondered if I meant that; I really did not want to go. Ignorance is bliss. I waited until my trip was over, the end of March 2000.

CHAPTER EIGHT

"When a door closes, a window flies open; key is, you have to find the breeze from that window."

Or for an alternate point of view, as Ms. Dorothy Parker once wrote:

"My land is bare of chattering folk, the clouds are low along the ridges, and sweet's the air with curly smoke from all my burning bridges."—*Sanctuary*

My heart and life prescription read: slow down. The opportunity came one day in late February 2000 when Mark, the practice owner, was at the clinic doing the surgery. This freed me to see the heavy client load for the day. The staff helped me clear the appointments that morning and I realized the time had arrived to make a move.

Letting go of my comfortable present had its benefits, like rest. The downside, though, could be a loss of a friend and a good income. I had to do this; there was no longer a choice. Walking into surgery, I shut the door behind me. Mark looked up from his work and smiled.

"All done?"

"Yep, they're cleared out and the staff is going to lunch."

"Good, we'll go in a minute."

I had to do this now. Mark would probably leave before

lunch and it would be days before I would see him again. Using the cabinet as a prop, I took a deep breath.

The words just fell out of my mouth, shattering to the floor. The clattering created an eerie fog of Dorothy's smoke in my mind, with a picture of my bridge of glass collapsing over our heads and landing around my feet and sending shards of an unexpected event into Mark's reality.

"Mark, I guess I just need to say it. I am resigning effective the end of March."

Mark jerked his head up, his stern blue eyes staring right at me. He seemed to turn white. My stomach was in knots; adrenaline was rushing through this conversation on both sides of the table.

"Why?" Mark asked, in his typically controlled and understated manner. His eyes gave his real thoughts away.

"Mark, I am not well. I am exhausted and I just cannot do this anymore!"

How could he not have seen this coming for the last few months? I had mentioned several times about clients asking me not to leave. Mark had even had a heads-up the year before.

Mark has historically gone to see an intuitive every three years or so. He was always seeking information about staff changes and economic trends. On his visit, about a year before this day, I had made a query of the intuitive for fun. During the course of the conversation with Mark, my name was mentioned.

"Janet is not well." The intuitive said no more than that single phrase.

Maybe Mark did not really listen to so much of what was said in reference to me that day. Hearing the tape Mark made of the visit, I stepped back when I heard the statement but even I blew it off.

Mark finished closing the incision, ripped off his mask,

cap, gloves and gown. Shane came in and recovered the animal from its state of sleep. Mark turned back to me.

"Let's walk back to radiology so we can talk."

Radiology was a grand word for a 4 x 8 room full of filing cabinets, radiographs, tables, tubes and processing equipment. It was dark (nice cover for facial reactions), and out of hearing range from others in the clinic. We sat at our opposing ends of the table. I was creating a schism and Mark was calculating a resolution.

"What about a couple of days a week? Janet, I need more notice than a month."

Mark was desperate to keep someone in that particular clinic. The spring was coming, this practice was very busy and had historically been hard to staff because of that factor. Mark had been good to me and I hated to have to leave, but as my Mom has been known to say, "Circumstances alter cases." They sure altered this one.

"No, Mark, I need to go, I'm not well. I need to slow down. I have to find out what is wrong with me. It's medical, Mark, not personal! I cannot drive these miles anymore, nor work the hours. I'm sorry, Mark; a month is the best I can do."

I knew in my heart that if I continued on there at any level, my life was only going to put me deeper in debt with my health. I stood, didn't look back and left the room. Mark was behind me, still trying to resolve this to his benefit.

"Think about working a couple of days a week at least."

The staff was standing in the treatment area and with those words knew I was leaving. Mark confirmed this,

"Janet may still work with us a couple of days a week."

That hopeful request fell on deaf ears for the cord that tied me mentally to the practice was severed. Losing an entire association with Mark was not the goal, but I felt I had done just that in that one brief moment. He would stew on this episode a while before reconciling the reasons for my leaving.

The last month of employment passed in what seemed a moment. I said goodbye to old clients and newfound friends, telling them only that I had decided to find a job closer to home. I did not speak with Mark again until after I knew my fate.

His attitude and that of the others in the clinic then appeared to change from one of betrayal to one of understanding. The only reason I had so drastically altered my behavior was the stress of the disease. They understood and accepted my reality, finally understanding the why of the difference they had seen over the years.

It really had nothing to do with them, or the job; it was all about me and the hell that my disease had brought into the picture. I was grateful they had the grace to readmit me to their fold, if only for the occasional get-together.

CHAPTER NINE

"Be true to your work, your word and your friend."
Thoreau

Focus shifted to the yearly Continuing Education trip with my friends. Every year, Dr. Ann, Dr. Traci and I would go to a national meeting. These meetings are designed to help veterinarians meet state requirements to maintain licensure to practice. It was to both learn and play. We always chose somewhere we had never been and made the most of the time. We had been to Reno, Chicago and now Toronto. This trip was going to be different though; it was overshadowed by my uncertain future.

My last appointment with Dr. Evans ended and the medical conversations began in my brain, trying to figure out what kind of mess I had gotten myself into this time. I was really sick, and not just with some minor little deal that would be gone in a couple of weeks. When Dr. Evans said there were immature white cells circulating in my blood stream, all I could think was leukemia. I tried not to diagnose myself since I had not seen the numbers. Supposing based on facts not in evidence (one of Becky's favorite phrases) would find no profit.

Inside my little pea-brain head, the procrastinator me kept saying, "Go on your trip, Janet; deal with it later." Only too eager to oblige that little voice, I packed my bags, boarded the plane and flew to Toronto.

Dr.Traci and I had become friends while in school. We had studied together and had run with the same crowd. We had worked together. So, it was easy yet very hard to tell her I was sick. But I had to tell someone not in my family. Too little information was available at this stage and my heart told me it was too soon for setting the family into action around this disease.

One evening near the end of our trip, Ann decided to rest. Traci and I didn't want to disturb her so we went downstairs to have a drink and talk. Walking into the hotel restaurant bar we were shown to a booth next to the window. Our waiter busily re-wiped the tabletop and handed us a menu.

"Ladies. Good evening. What can I get for you? We have martinis on special tonight."

It was later in the evening and though not really wanting a drink, I ordered a blue sapphire anyway. Traci decided on a cosmopolitan. We agreed to share a fruit and cheese plate.

The bar was decorated in a very dark manner: dark wood, dark appointments, just dark. Even though full, the air was heavy with quiet. My day had been spent working on the structure of a sentence to let Traci in on what an undecided future I was facing. The right words would not crystallize into a sentence that made any sense and that also represented my present state of "unknowing."

In that moment, sitting in a Toronto hotel bar, after a long day of learning, I was dreadfully aware of my dying. I needed to hear that fact spoken out loud, to share it with someone who knew me and would understand exactly what those words meant. Fortunately or unfortunately for Traci, she was it. So, being the blunt person I am on occasion, I just blurted it out; no need to pussyfoot, especially around this issue.

"Traci, I'm sick. I might have a leukemia."

I paused, sat back in my chair, picked up my drink, took a good sip, lifted my eyes to Traci and waited for a reaction. The warm alcohol slipped down my throat and burned like fire just as my words hit their target hard. Traci jerked back from the table deep into her seat and looked at me with the eyes of both a doctor and a frightened friend.

"What do you mean? Why do you say that? What kind?"

She kept staring at me, impatient for a response.

"I don't know. All I have are CBC results."

I told her the heart doctor saga and what Dr. Evans had found before I left town.

"They say I need a hem/onc."

Not wanting to see the worry in my friend's eyes, I just stared into my glass of warming blue martini. I don't think two pitchers of Martinis could have made a dent in the emotional charge running through me. Might as well let it sit and get hot.

"Why?"

Traci was digging but she was calm.

"I have a left shift, very left shift without infection, all cell lines. Remember, a doctor had seen something similar while I was still in Mobile. He wanted me to go then to a hematologist. I didn't, because he thought it was a drug response and not a leukemia and I did not want to spend the money out of my pocket for his interest. I don't know, maybe I should have."

I was fading out of a conversation that was too hard to utter as well as too hard to hear. Besides, it was Traci's turn to chew on those uncluttered words for a while. Picking up a grape and rolling it between my fingers, watching the blue color of my drink reflect into the tears of moisture running down the pitcher and onto the tablecloth, Traci's reaction brought me back to the discussion.

"Well, Jan, just wait until you know; it could be a number of things. We will be there for you whatever you find. I'll say a novena for you. I say them for David; they always work. I cannot imagine that both you and David have bone marrow disease. How likely is that?"

Traci seemed to wander off mentally for a moment and then took a sip of her drink. She again looked away, not wanting me to see the small tear that had crept along her lower eyelid and down her cheek. I had just witnessed the first of many tears and worried looks to come with this tale.

"Thanks, Traci, I appreciate your prayers. I really don't want to eat this stuff, do you? I'm tired; let's go."

We left our warm martinis and half-eaten platter of food in that dark Toronto bar and walked to the elevator. The ride back up was silent except for the closing door and whirring motor of the car as it traveled the distance to our floor. Ann had already fallen asleep.

I did not tell Ann about my illness on that trip. Her mother was dying and I did not want to tell her bad news to add to what she already had to deal with daily. I think I did not tell her the whole story until right before our trip to Boston the next year. Ann's mom died the year of this Toronto trip in July 2000.

CHAPTER TEN

"Never fear the shadows. They simply mean there's a light shining somewhere nearby."

Ruth E. Renkel

In the beginning of April 2000, a new job demanded and needed all loose ends tidied up. Appointments were made and all yearly trips to doctors and dentists were finished, all except going to the oncologist. I just revisited my G.P. There was a promise to repeat the blood tests.

The vampire's office opened early one morning, my allotted donation of blood was removed and I bolted out the door, leaving any thought of my future health at the clinic. Well, at least until the results came back.

Dr. Tom Evans has cared for my health nearly all of my life. He is a quiet man, large, an ex-athlete, and a father of two. He is jovial, intelligent, not given to hype and available. A few days after the blood-letting had passed I was called to come back for the results. I was sitting on the exam table when Tom bolted through the door. He made one comment.

"Alright, Janet, now you have nucleated red cells peripherally. You are not going to put this off any longer!"

The jig was up. Dr. Tom had spoken. Immature white cells had been in my blood stream for some time; but the shift to include immature red cells was the clincher. This disease could no longer be ignored. Presence was a requirement; give up the procrastination, Janet, give in to the demand. This blood anomaly was real. The dog bite had healed long ago; no more excuses.

Relief ruled the day; responsibility to my health became the goal. Dr. Tom referred the case to Dr. Tracy Dobbs at Baptist Hospital in Knoxville.

CHAPTER ELEVEN

"A cheerful heart is good medicine."

Proverbs 17:22 NIV

Tracy Dobbs is a clean cut, nice-looking, well-dressed, friendly, communicative, capable doctor. He is straightforward, a wonderfully compassionate person. Those characteristics did not make my visit less unnerving. Blood work was completed and my first bone marrow tap and an abdominal CT were to be scheduled for the next week. Dobbs had said my spleen seemed enlarged.

Dr. Dobbs assessed my blood tests during this first visit, and he mentioned the terms chronic myelogenous leukemia, or CML, and acute myelogenous leukemia, or AML. That office visit left me with a pervading numbness or maybe a disconnection from the process. A detour was created so that this visit could move away from the path it was moving toward. I wanted to stop it from moving forward into my consciousness. I soon found myself empathizing with a cat in my exam room. I felt like a cat that quickly hides its head in its owner's abdomen, just knowing that if he couldn't see me, I couldn't see him, so his reality was the truth. I just knew that if I could not mentally see what had just occurred I would be fine.

Regardless of the tried mental gymnastics to stay the progress of this possibility, my final recognition was that my body and I were not looking forward to the next few weeks' activities. A bad case of uncertainty and anticipation followed the visit.

Sometimes I wished I had not known so much medicine. I was feeling rather in awe of my dilemma in that moment. The mere 35 miles home took an eternity and the road swept by with no recognized landmarks. Pulling into the drive late that day, even my home seemed hauntingly different from the one that I had left that morning.

The Fleming-Smith home in Rockwood was constructed in the late 1800s for my greatgrandfather, Dr. Isaac G. Fleming. The house is large, two-story, Victorian in architecture, with a wrap-around porch, gingerbread in the peaks of the roof, shutters on the windows, wood floors, and no closets. I am the fourth generation to live under its roof. Our home is a grand old haunted home, full of history and family continuity. I love the house for all of those reasons. That particular afternoon, though, I looked at my home through the eyes of a dying person. My heart ached and I fought back the tears of the potential and real loss the day's news had brought to its door.

I opened the car door, got out, took a deep, yet stilted breath, swallowed my tears, gathered my thoughts, my courage, and then said a prayer that God would direct my words. Walking through the front door, meeting the dogs, as usual, I wandered into the kitchen with my cocker spaniels, Topper and Heather, racing around behind the heels of my feet.

My loving, little 82-year-old mother (who had just four brief years earlier lost her husband of 46 years) was standing there in the doorway with fear all over her face.

Mom's shoulders were rounded, her chest was caved in, and her hands, still wearing the rings my father had given her, were wrapped around themselves. The kitchen, the scene of so many family joys and crises had one more tale to tell. She stood there, looking at her eldest daughter with her frightened blue eyes, and as I looked back at her I spoke in a voice that seemed to come from somewhere else.

"Your daughter might have a leukemia," I said, immediately wishing I could pull the words back into my mouth and delete them from our life.

Why did I say anything to her without knowing all the facts? It would have been so easy to say they did not know anything yet. But she was my mom and she was frightened and concerned. She, of all people, deserved to know what I knew when I knew it.

Mom, her face sagging with the news and in true form, did not say much. She did not have to; she hugged me as if I would disappear. This was not the time for tears or fears of what might be. I did not have the luxury of mind games at this moment. I needed a clear mind to deal with the decisions I would be required to make in the next year.

CHAPTER TWELVE

"Keep trusting; there is a plan."

Having found a new job before the test results had come back, I was hoping that job would still be mine. The work contract at the new place was not yet final, an intentional move on my part until I knew what disease I was facing. The day after visiting Dr. Dobbs I walked into work thinking it would be my last.

"Doc, may I speak with you in private?"

"Sure, let's go in the office."

We closed the door.

"I might be very ill and it will be a few weeks before I know the outcome. Since we have not finalized the contract I wanted to give you an opportunity to back out if you wanted."

I was not expecting to keep the same agreement. I was sick and probably not going to be as dependable. Not knowing how this still unknown disease would play out over the next year, honesty had to be the best route.

"I thought something was unsaid earlier. Don't worry; it's not a problem. We can continue with the contract."

"Thank you, Doc. One other point: I do not feel comfortable in telling any of the clinic staff. I don't know for sure and I really do not want others to know yet."

The need to protect myself from the curiosity of others at this moment was paramount.

"Fine, but you should tell them."

"I will, but not yet."

We walked out of the office to a crowd of people standing around and staring. They knew something had happened; I did not want them to know what had happened.

When people know you are sick, they treat you differently. I did not want to be treated differently. Starting a new job and building new relationships required an even playing field, not one altered by their perception of my disease. Life was going to change in monumental ways soon enough, and those changes would make others realize my lack of health.

I went to work trying to leave my illness at the door each morning, not wanting to make the same mistakes I had made at my previous job. I was mindful of that fact every day. That choice made my stress level a little greater, but it had to be done.

Early on, the decision was made to not tell my siblings what calamity was unfolding in my life. Mom knew not to talk to them about my situation; this was my news to tell in my own way and time. Why prematurely worry them and create more stress for myself by having to deal with questions for which I had no answer?

Soon after my initial visit to Dr. Dobbs, my cousin Mary and her husband Don brought their cat, Sam, in to see me at the clinic. Mary, my mother's niece, helped raise me and my siblings. There is not a time I do not remember Mary being there as we grew up. She lived with us one summer when we lived in Houston. She taught me to skate, to drive a car, she led the way career-wise and became a chemist. She married a research chemist. Mary was more my older sister than a cousin. After she married Don, he too became an integral part of our lives. They could know but only with the caveat.

I closed the door. "I have some bad news and I don't want my siblings to know until I have an answer."

Mary spoke back, "What? OK, we won't say anything."

"I'm sick. I may have a leukemia of some sort."

Their faces said it all. Don was crestfallen. His eyes showed how unbelievably hard my words had smashed into their lives. Mary ran over and hugged me.

"Oh, Janet."

Her voice sounded of fear and the compassion one can count on from Mary.

"Janet, you should tell your siblings; let them be there for you."

I knew Mary was right, my siblings would be, but I had other plans.

"No, I am not going to let them worry anymore than they have to. When I know what I have, I will tell them."

"Janet you should let them help you through the wait."

Mary was certain I should tell them all.

"No. I have decided when I know for sure I will tell them."

I knew their knowledge of my crisis would send them into constant phone calls, pushing me to seek answers to questions that I did not have the information to even pose for myself. I did not need that right now.

"Okay."

Mary and Don met the caveat. It was nice to have them in the loop. My dependence on others was to grow soon to unbelievable levels. Beginning that behavior cycle with Mary and Don would make the future need requirements more palatable. I am an independent old cuss, as are all Smiths, and learning to depend totally on others would be a major lesson.

I persisted in not telling my siblings until I knew the results. Mother, Mary, Don and I dealt with the unknown alone. Having said that, there was an incident that almost "ratted" me out of the silence.

One sunny afternoon Mom and I were sitting at the kitchen table having a cup of hot tea when the phone rang. I got up walked across the kitchen and picked up.

"Hello?"

"Hey, Sis, are you feeling alright? Is your heart OK?" It was Becky.

My younger sister, Becky, has always had a sixth sense about family members. Knowing I had gone to a cardiologist and that I had an arrhythmia, she spoke as if she knew something was not quite right in Rockwood.

I, in good conscience, said, "It's just fine. The drug doesn't seem to help much though."

"Okay, is Rosebud doing alright?"

"Yeah, Mom's fine"

"Alright, then, are you sure?"

"Yes Sis, I'm sure."

"I'll talk to you later then, bye."

Becky hung up; I looked at Mom.

"That Becky, she knows everything!"

I did not mention my blood. She did not ask. Many months after this conversation she mentioned, "I'll dig deeper the next time I ask after your health!"

Those initial test results and their implications had rocked my world. Those tentacles would invade the lives of the people who loved me soon enough.

CHAPTER THIRTEEN

"No test or temptation that comes your way is beyond the course of what others had had to face. All you need remember is that God will never let you down; He will never let you be pushed past your limit; He'll always be there to help you come through it."

1 Corinthians 10:3 MSG

The following week, because I would require sedation for the testing, Don drove me into Knoxville for the bone marrow tap and the abdominal CT. My mind was creating sensations of pain and enlarging the uncertainty around the day's activity. Treks off into the possibilities in this unknown world of disease would create mental monsters for a while.

I had completed a bone marrow tap on animals a time or two but knowing how to do one and having one done to you is another rung up the reality ladder. Honestly, it is the worst. My mind's eye saw a medically correct and quite graphic color illustration of each tissue breached during the procedure and what would happen to that tissue as the needle tore through it, headed for my inner sanctum of survival, the bone marrow.

Mind, turn off; please. Just get through this day and it will be done, life will go on, pain will subside. I opened the door and found that the hem/onc office at Baptist was a busy place. Walking through the door I nearly fell into the lap of a man in a wheelchair. I hadn't even noticed him. I apologized as he laughed.

The office was one of those wall-papered, brightly lit, overstuffed chair kind of waiting rooms. There was the obligatory friendly staff and a typical view of downtown Knoxville and the Tennessee River; strangely comforting. I signed the check-in sheet and confirmed my insurance information.

Unwilling voyeur, unsettled observer and patient, I sat in a chair full of porcupine needles and fidgeted to get comfortable as I watched other people in various stages of cancer treatment travel in and out of the door. Don sat down and found a magazine. The door across the room opened.

"Dr. Janet?"

Having just sat down to my uncomfortable view, I stood on floors that seemed to offer no support and followed the nurse into the hallway. She placed me on the scale, wrote down my weight, 147 pounds, and then we walked into the lab area.

A high-traffic area, the lab was an L-shaped room full of blood analyzers, printers, blinking lights and buzzing machines, busy nurses and doctors traveling in and out of the door. Orders flew around the room like confetti during Mardi Gras.

"Hi, Dr. Janet, have a seat and we'll draw your blood. How ya' feeling?" The nurse was a fellow Roane Countian.

"A little nervous, but OK."

I sat in the lab chair and rolled up my sleeve. She took my blood pressure and my blood. Sitting in that hard lab chair I watched the analyzer tick off my white count and waited for the results, hoping for some rewind to the time when they were all normal. It did not happen. The values were still very abnormal, worse actually. My bone marrow had developed a mind of its own by now, and I was praying it was something we could rein in again, as if an errant child or young horse.

"Dr. Janet?" A new nurse spoke my name, breaking my focus from the count. "Come this way and we will get you ready for the tap."

We walked across the hall and into a larger room. Rather than white or green, it was painted in a pale creamy yellow. Windows were all along one wall, hung with yellow checked curtains and, again, the Tennessee River was visible. Spring was on the way and early flower colors were counting themselves present all along the river bank. I could view dogwoods and redbuds, a few jonquils and tulips, something nice to look at while I waited for the tissue tearing.

The lab table was in the center of the room. A yellow checked curtain divided the space into half. My heart was racing and my breathing was becoming noticeably faster, my personal exhaust heating air already heavy with growing fear of the procedure to come and the unknown life that waited for me with the results.

My mind was working overtime and a reality that would carry me through this ordeal was surfacing. I had to get my thoughts back in line with truth, and the known facts, not in fearing the unknown or in guessing. There would be no profit in fear and supposing.

The nurse spoke again.

"Dr. Janet, you will need to lie on this table on your left side when we do the tap. Let me put an I.V. catheter in your hand."

She prepped the vein area, pushed the stylet through my skin and into the large vein on top of my hand. I felt a pop through the skin, and a pop as the catheter entered into my vein. My skin only stung a moment, the vein not at all. She finished the placement. I lowered my slacks below my hip bones and lay down on the table.

"OK, on your side."

She placed a sheet over my hips and legs.

"I am going to get the site prepped, it will feel cold."

I was already shaking inside, so what if the cold made it worse? About that time, Dr. Dobbs walked in, smiling, as usual.

"Hello Janet."

Did you give her any sedative?"

"No, not yet."

"Well, she might need one since this is the first tap; it may help with some of the anxiety. What do you think Janet?"

"Sure, my mind seems to want to run wild with this. I don't quite know what to expect."

They lowered their voices and were speaking now as if I were not there. I found I was not thinking about the procedure, instead I was sensing a new definition of Janet Smith, DVM, pushing its unwanted way into my unassuming little life.

The nurse gave me the injection; I relaxed, closed my eyes and faintly heard Dr. Dobbs begin to talk me through the procedure. First, he injected the tap site on my pelvis with lidocaine.

"This will burn for just a second, and then we will be ready. I am making an incision now, Janet. I am inserting the needle. You may feel pressure when I pull the plunger back. Done. Janet, they will put a pressure bandage on the site, leave it on until tomorrow. I will see you in two to three weeks and we will discuss what we find. Any questions?"

There was no reply to his question because the effect of the Valium still controlled all of my reactions. Dr. Dobbs stepped back from the table.

"OK, I will see you in a couple of weeks. Call if you need anything."

The anticipation of the procedure and the mental demons surrounding the unknown were again worse than the reality of the tap. This lesson of realizing that my mind's eye of a situation was always worse than the reality of it was finally starting to sink in.

The nurse placed a pressure bandage that I was to leave alone for 24 hours on my tap site and then sent me down for my CT. I drank my opaque liquid; 20 minutes inside the CT scanner and I was finished. Don met me in the waiting room and we headed home.

"You OK, kid?"

"Yeah, I'm OK, just a little sleepy."

A poor reply to a heartfelt question. We drove home in relative silence, for my thoughts were whirling in my brain. The week before Dr. Dobbs and I had had a long discussion on CML and the ramifications the disease carried.

I was sitting on the exam table. Dr. Dobbs was on a chair at its foot. He spoke with seriousness, but without being alarmist.

"Janet, I just wanted to go over this with you one more time and make sure you know what we are talking about here. CML is only one of the diseases you could have. It's the horse, not the zebra. CML is the most likely, based on initial results, but we won't know until the marrow is read."

I know. What does CML do to the marrow?"

My scientific background was driving me to fact, not feeling. I needed the human aspect of this marrow disease. Humans, though mammals, react differently to disease with the same variability as different species do in vet medicine. I only wanted facts that would allow me the insight to deal with this journey. Maybes, what ifs, and we'll sees were not going to give me the strength to make choices. I hoped my doctors would understand this about me.

"Well, it is insidious, chronic; that is good in that there is some time. At first, your white count will rise because you produce too many white cells. Eventually the other cell lines decrease in count. You could become anemic. The white cells don't function properly so you can get infections. Eventually, the platelets drop and you can bleed. The progression can result in an acute onset of the leukemia. This is most often a terminal event."

"If it is CML, is there any treatment?"

I didn't want to hear him give this answer. The answer was already in my mind. Why could I not shut my brain off?

"No, not really. We can try to modulate it with drugs like interferon and hydrea and a new drug called Gleevec is showing some promise. Sometimes transplants work."

"Sounds lovely."

"Yeah, it is serious, but until we know for sure don't dwell on this too much, OK?"

"Sure, I will try not to see too many demons at my door. Thanks, and bye, Doc."

My mind was working overtime, questioning how it would be CML. My red count was very immature and rising, not falling. My platelets were up, not down. I had a feeling he was protecting me from something, I didn't know what. His admonition not to dwell landed on deaf ears. How could I not dwell on it now that the horse was out of the barn?

A black horse named "Future" was spooked and seemed well on his way to the land of the dying. Unfortunately, that frantic horse had me on its back, clinging to his mane for support while traveling at a full gallop, him totally unresponsive to any aid I gave to slow his gait.

Getting up, I felt my knees go out from under me if only for a second and I wandered to the check-out desk, scheduled my next appointment, and left.

CHAPTER FOURTEEN

> "The more I work with the body, keeping my assumptions in a temporary state of reservation, the more I appreciate and sympathize with a given "disease." The body no longer appears as a sick or irrational demon, but as a process with its own inner logic and wisdom."
>
> Dr. Thomas Arnold Mindell

Time passed slowly during the three weeks of waiting for the bone marrow and CT test results. The new job was a joy. The pace was much slower and the duties shared, happy to not be spending so much of life in an automobile. The clinic staff worked hard and had a lot of fun in between clients. The job kept my mind from pursuing the possibilities of my day for revelation.

Dobbs kept office hours in Roane County one morning a week, a short drive from my home. About 10:30 I was put in an exam room, small, but comfortable. To say I was terrified going into that room would have truly been the definition of understatement. I felt my future walk out as I walked through that door.

The room had a sink, a single cabinet, a chair and an exam table. Seems odd how observing my environment still took on such importance. I guess I knew I was going to be in that environment for a while so I might as well learn how to cope.

Sitting on that exam table waiting for Dr. Dobbs, I noticed my heart was revving up for the meeting and I was shivering as if freezing. Surreal feelings flooded my senses, and just as quickly the perception of my surroundings became very hazy and far away.

Then the door swung open. The nurse strolled in, smiling.

"Good morning, Dr. Smith, how are you?"

"Fine, yourself?" I lied.

"Doing well, thank-you."

She took my blood pressure and temperature and turned to face me.

"Dr. Smith, do you have hypertension? Your blood pressure is 150/90."

A nice pat answer that seemed to cover a multitude of patient symptoms came in my response.

"No, just nervous, wanting the wait over, I guess."

She smiled back at me, shook her head as if she understood and spoke on her way out.

"Dr. Dobbs will be right with you."

Once again sitting alone in that room, there was only the quiet of eternity. The air was motionless yet pressing, stale and powerfully present. A wisp of that stale scent became recognizable, the same sulfur odor I recognized in Dr. Bishop's office that day, fear of my future or lack of one.

I had never feared the future before. I had always figured any change needed to come, even if I had fought it at first. I usually embraced new opportunity. This day brought no trappings of opportunity, or it did not seem like it at the time.

This day was morphing into a black hole. A black hole whose overpowering vacuum was trying to suck the sense out of me and its hope snuffing gravitational power needed to be avoided and escaped. Focusing on some inane activity, filling my mind with nonsense, giving this creation of my mind no room to grow any larger could stop the encroachment long enough to get my answer.

So, I sat on that cold exam table; waiting on my future to walk in the door. I waited all alone. I fidgeted with outdated magazines, tore the paper on the table, scanned the room as if daring any obvious change in the fabric of my life to appear in that moment of waiting. I then turned my efforts to running song lyrics through my head and waited some more.

Another eternity passed through all that fidgeting. I nervously popped my leg up and down upon the step at the foot of the exam table, setting the table into motion and into a harmonic state equal to the shaking of my insides. I just wanted, no, desperately needed, to get this session over. I needed the truth; I always have.

Stressed to the max, two thoughts could not form in my head; even the song lyrics were messing up. Having put my brain into standby, with all the movement and mental recitations, I finally zoned out. That mental state was a blessing! Calm was all I felt. I needed to remember how I got there. My "foe", fear, was so palpably close to permanently moving into my psyche. I needed to know my fate. Exposure of the cause of my fear would free me and fear would no longer have any hold on my future. Fear would only leave when I had that answer.

Still I did not want to hear it. My life as I knew it was only moments away from extinction. I had worked my lifetime to find this existence and in a heartbeat, with a single word, my existence would be gone.

In that moment of recognition, I prayed for God's grace, shamelessly begging Him to grant me the strength to deal with

Dobbs' answer. The facts were easy; it was the unknowing that was ripping my seams at this moment. I kept reminding my pitiful little mind that the fear would pass as the knowledge would give me power. I had to believe my own dogma. As a scientist, I knew facts would create a path through the uncertainty.

Hearing a voice, I realized Dr. Dobbs was outside my exam room door on the phone, speaking with the lab about my bone marrow results. Seems I was eavesdropping but it was my own information; I felt entitled to hear the conversation. Not boding well for me, I thought. Why did he have to call for the result at this late date? Had the lab messed up? Was the sample non-diagnostic? Would I have to have another tap? Or was it something unexpected like those in the zebra line? I focused on Dobbs' voice again. His tenor changed.

"Really? No kidding? Are you sure?"

With those few questions I knew something very different was coming. Being one who had dealt with pathologists, I knew a zebra when I heard those hoof-beats.

Dobbs walked in the door; his usually smiling face was hidden as his head was down, his skin was flushed and even he was fidgeting; he, with my medical file. In my heart I knew he was searching for the right words to gently place me further along the path into my uncertain future. At least I hoped I had a future.

My heart sank, suddenly very afraid of what he was going to tell me. I felt like that proverbial wild animal standing in the road, having been hit with headlights. I knew that car was coming, I wanted to run, but the need to know overrode the fear. After all, Janet, was this not what the last few weeks and months had been about? Truth had to be faced. Take a deep breath; grab the edge of the table and "buck up, sister."

Dobbs moved to the front of the exam table, sat on the stool at its foot, looked at me, dropped his head, and then delivered the news that would occupy my life and the lives of those around me for some time to come. He took that deep breath, raised his eyes to mine and the words came stumbling out of his mouth. Quietly, compassionately and thoughtfully the diagnosis we were searching for came in one long word.

"Janet, you have myelofibrosis, a rare one."

Blast those zebras! I knew it was going to be weird.

Dr. Dobbs searched my blank face for a reaction. I shut him out, narrowed my eyelids and allowed my Rolodex mind to busily flip through my mental vocabulary of medical terms while simultaneously revisiting pathology slides in my mind's eye, busily developing the disease in words and pictures. Retrieve: bone marrow pathology. Searching for a scientific peg to grab onto so to intelligently react to his words. I was busy! I was being a medical person, running consequences of that term and its definition in relation to what, where, cause, effect, treatment, prognosis. It seemed minutes had passed in the few seconds my mind had needed to generate the information to fully understand that term. Then it hit me.

Myelofibrosis, AMM, agnogenic myeloid metaplasia; I knew that term, and not by all of the human designations. I start shaking my head in understanding and spoke.

"In veterinary medicine we see it in cats with feline leukemia virus, occasionally in dogs. It is a rare bird with us also. We also refer to it as myleopthistic disease."

Dobbs shook his head in agreement and spoke again, very low in tone and somber.

"Janet, you know that fibrosis compresses the bone marrow with fibrocytes that start multiplying, that they scar the bone marrow down so that it no longer exists as a functioning organ. Janet, the CT shows that your spleen is enormous."

Tracy had put my file down and was leaning forward, trying to make sure I understood what he had told me. I had heard him loud and penetrating, like one of Cissy's farm calls. Like one of those farm calls, my response was as a child caught doing something they should not be doing. My core was quaking and I was trying to justify what was happening to my life.

"Janet, lie back and let me palpate your spleen again."

I lay back on the table and loosened my waistline and began a journey into myself. My past was all too logical now. Symptoms I had had for years finally made sense, making the picture of my disease state all too clear.

Years of my spleen working in overdrive, trying to clean up my blood and trying to create normal blood cells, had expanded itself into a huge space-occupying mass. It now covered an area the length of my abdomen from diaphragm to pelvis, and it filled over half of the width of that cavity. Normally, the spleen is a few inches long and wide and weighs a few ounces.

No wonder my digestive system was a mess. My stomach and bowel, mashed into the narrow space left in my abdomen, had nowhere to expand. No wonder I could not eat without pain and such severe heartburn, was so exhausted, and why, despite my weight loss of 20 pounds, my abdomen still appeared as if I were five or six months pregnant. No wonder I could not take a shower without itching all over, typical with myeloproliferative disease.

"Spleen baby," as I and my family came to call this huge organ, came out of hiding, and I could not wait until it was "born" and out of me! I had been peri-menopausal since my mid-thirties. Severe mood swings were my constant companion. I was now menopausal at the age of 47. I wondered if this disease had not pushed this biological hurdle along more quickly as well.

Dobbs broke the silence.

"OK, you can sit up now, Janet."

He sat back down on the stool and continued the conversation.

"Janet, are you doing OK? Do you want me to go on right now?"

"Yes." I waved my hands in the air, signaling his right to continue. "I'm OK; let's just get this over with."

"The disease has been there a long time, in all likelihood. So there is some good news around that fact. Your hemoglobin is still normal. Even your white count is not too elevated, and your platelets are still in a lower range where you shouldn't need medication to try to reduce their counts."

Dobbs spoke again.

"Janet, unfortunately, there is no medicine that will cure this disease. The only possible cure is a bone marrow transplant, or stem cell transplant. Some people try to slow it down with interferon, but it is a hard drug to tolerate and I feel it should be a drug of last recourse. There is also some concept that interferon may inhibit the ability of a transplant to engraft. Hydroxyurea is another drug that some people have tried. It too may inhibit engraftment. Transplant is a procedure we will not consider until there is no other route. It is truly life and death at that stage of the disease. We will not rush that choice."

Dr. Dobbs had finished his initial read of the problem.

Dobbs watched me closely for a reaction. I am afraid I was too numb to be very responsive. I knew about all of the drugs; we use them in vet med too. I was there, but "I" was gone.

The major immediate downside was my living with this knowledge daily, knowing a certain set of circumstances would dictate the timing of the medical activity. My doctors, correctly, were in no hurry to rush me into a situation in which such high risk of loss of life was inherent.

This was the end of May 2000; I was 47 years old. I was going to die if I did nothing and could die if I did act. The next question: when would I face this ultimate choice? Time was my controller; this disease loved time.

I found, though, that time was also to be my first gift of grace: time to deal with my looming mortality. I had been dying: year by year, day by day and now, abruptly, second by second. I knew what 24 hours before I had been ignorant of. I only had moments now, not years. How could I come to terms with what I had left undone? How could I face my death when I had not really faced my own life?

The soul-searching began; the quest was in overdrive and I wanted to go into autopilot, the easy path to shut-down. Really, the shift into catatonia might be nice for the next few years. Catatonia in comparison, though, would be way too easy and selfish. My family should not be burdened with someone who would not meet this situation head-on. This was my life, what was left of it; I had to be present. I was soon realizing being present was not going to be easy. Nothing about this situation was going to be easy.

CHAPTER FIFTEEN

"I don't know how to tell you, but...."

As I drove home with the diagnosis hanging over me, my realization became obvious. The siblings were now in the place of need to know. Their lives were going to be drastically impacted by this illness. That day the phone calls began, from me to them, from them to each other. Odd, but I don't remember how I told each of them the diagnosis. I called Becky first, then Jack, because I knew how scared Becky would be and would need to talk to him about the change facing our lives. He lives in Atlanta, as does Becky. I then called Laura in Maryland. Laura had Rick to turn to for comfort and being a nurse she would understand most of the medicine.

Lastly, I called Larry, my brother, the doctor. I needed to really talk to Larry for a long time about the mess in which I had found myself living. He would know what I was facing and where I needed to go to find answers. He took the news with a heavy heart but well. While talking to me that evening, he told me of his friend, a hematologist there in Gainesville.

"Janet, I'd trust this guy with my family's life; come down and talk to Bruce." I did not respond except, "We'll see."

In that moment, I did not need more outside information. I needed to let Dobbs' words quietly flow like a meandering creek through my body; they needed to eddy and bubble in my brain, and seep into my consciousness word by unbelievable word, where the pressure of their presence would send them spewing from my mouth. I needed to feel this knowledge within me. The spewing of that verbal confirmation to others reminded me that this was not a dream, even though it felt like a night-fright. The only other words I needed to hear were those of support and love from my family.

The siblings all did well with the disease when around me; it was when they were not with me that the prospect took its toll. Jack, who has a very difficult time with medical impacts on his family, told Becky, "I just can't get my arms around this."

Becky agreed.

I was having quite a hard time getting my own arms around this problem. The immensity of the consequences of this disease seemed overwhelming. So many aspects of my life and my family's life would be altered. If I died, someone would have to really change their life in that Mother would need something different than what she had with me still in the world. Eventually though, time and focused meditation brought ways to get my arms around my new reality and more.

CHAPTER SIXTEEN

"We don't receive wisdom, we must discover it for ourselves after a journey that no one can take us or spare us."

Marcel Proust

Life changed for the better; the stressful job was gone and I knew what I was facing. I worked four-and-a-half days a week, taking naps on the table in radiology when clients were not present. Time at home found me reading about the disease process and searching for answers to my questions. I was in the science/doctor mode. I had become my own patient. The internet turned out to not be my friend.

Having gone through much information, I found it too broad and too unfiltered to help. I have never gone back to the net as a source of general medical information. The knowledge gained could create greater monsters in my mind than were true. Two members of my immediate family were in the medical field. They would become my source for medical information. Many questions still needed answers and even after all of the study, a certain level of fear of the unknown loomed large because each new source raised new unanswerable questions.

Every month brought another visit to Dr. Dobbs to follow the disease progress. The cell count results were still in a consistent place. Conversations turned to getting more information about transplant. There would be a need to locate a new doctor and hospital because Baptist did not do transplants.

The start of the search for a donor needed to begin so there would be time to search the donor bank if none of my family matched. The enormity of that occurrence had not registered in my consciousness. To have ventured down that road at this moment would have been the suicide of hope. Dr. Dobbs had the plan formed at one of my visits to recheck my values.

"I want you to see Dr. Steven Wolff. Janet, Steve is a great doctor, really a bright guy, but be ready; he's a little hyper!" Dobbs was grinning.

"Sure, whatever you think is best."

Thus I lost my first doctor of the journey.

Experience teaches that sooner or later we will defer to the experts. Even though veterinary medicine laid a wonderful foundation for understanding the passage, it made the abdication of my responsibility to my medical state much more difficult. But this moment solidified the fact that I was not capable of dealing with this disease. Dobbs' releasing of my case to Vanderbilt made me realize that my letting go was all that was left on my plate in the medical realm. My plate was full of dealing with the life-altering implications of my disease. Only my doctor could direct this show.

Finally, I accepted what I had known and subverted from the beginning: that I needed to be the patient. I certainly had no clue where to go or who to see what to do next. I needed my doctor to point me in the right direction. I quit trying to do the medical work right then and there. I retired my computer and found that there was no shame in my need of becoming a sheep reacting to a shepherd. In a way, it was comforting.

I had this idea that my body had become a vessel carrying some weird parasite that would eat at my earthly fiber and methodically sink me when it could. In that moment, I resigned my captaincy over the USS Myeloid and took my sick little self to the sick bay. Let someone with the necessary experience and knowledge control the helm. Not my job anymore.

My job was the most important; my life depended on handling it to perfection. Circumstances dictated loving my family and surviving. If surviving this disease was not part of the plan, then giving this disease process a damn good run for the money was part of the plan. That was all I needed to worry about now.

My visits to see Dr. Dobbs would be only cursory after this move. I would miss his compassion and directness; he had served the search well and would continue to be there when I needed his help.

The hem/onc office at Baptist set up my first appointment at Vanderbilt University Medical Center, located in Nashville, Tennessee. The information interview with Dr. Steven Wolff, the head of the stem cell transplant program at VUMC, was set for July 5, 2000.

CHAPTER SEVENTEEN

"What's it all about, Dr. Steve?"

July fifth was a beautiful, bright summer day. My little Acura CL was cruising, the sunroof open and the CD player blaring Diana Krall's latest venture. The path to the future took I-40 West through Middle Tennessee. The route turned off I-40 onto the Broadway ramp, turned left and left again off West End split, then around to 21st straight down to Vanderbilt campus and then right into the hospital complex.

My first sight of Vanderbilt that day left an impression: overpowering and huge. Driving around the circle, looking up, I was lost in a tunnel of white crosswalks and 11 stories of hospital in red oxide brick. The edifice of Vanderbilt Hospital claimed either side of the street. Cars, patients, patients' families and visitors, doctors, nurses, aides, students, valets, police, ambulances, helicopters, insatiable action, interminable noise, construction everywhere was this entity called "Vanderbilt."

This was not the first time I had been to Vandy but I was a patient this time around. My great uncles had gotten their education in dentistry at Vanderbilt in the late 1800s and early 1900s. My cousin Gary earned his engineering degree at Vanderbilt. Don's niece, Betsy, graduated from Vanderbilt Medical School. Vandy was a place that had never been on my radar screen except for family ties. Vanderbilt was just a large university and hospital near downtown Nashville. A group of buildings I knew I would not need in my life.

Oops, guess I was wrong. On this day, VUMC became my place of hope. It was not bricks and mortar; it was a teeming source of medical knowledge, ability, compassion and my future. I looked at Vandy as a new lover looks at her amore: all the flaws and the unknowns were hidden. The bliss of ignorance once again pervaded my future.

I parked in the clinic garage and walked across the pedestrian bridge, wandering down the hall looking for room 2603. At a bend in the hall, I saw the sign, a glass wall and at ground level a fountain. Turning to the right the check-in desk was visible on the right. Vanderbilt had mailed a donor information packet to me before my visit, requesting I fill it out before seeing Dr. Wolff.

The receptionist looked up.

"May I help you?"

"Yes, I am Janet Smith. I have an appointment with Dr. Wolff."

She handed me papers to fill out and then she offered not a smile, only a question.

"Did you bring the donor information?"

"I have not filled it out. I want more information before I make a choice."

I looked her in the eye, standing my position of ignorance.

"The doctors like to have that information at your first visit."

"I understand that, but this may be my only visit." (Stubborn defiance is thy name, old girl.)

She was not too happy with me, her look of annoyance was obvious, but I needed to have some level of control in this process. I did not want to be bulldozed onto a road I had not consciously chosen. Medicine gets into an activity groove and before you know it things are happening at breakneck speed and you wonder what the heck happened. I did not want that experience. I realized she was busy, and probably tired, but I hoped not all interactions that day would be so abrupt and unpleasant.

Once checked in, I sat down in the waiting room and found myself quite uncomfortable; that porcupine needle-filled chair must have followed me from Knoxville. The people sitting around the room were waiting for their appointments. I soon realized I was in a room full of hope and possibility. I was in a room full of survivors!

These survivors were bald, were wearing masks, were in wheelchairs and still had catheter ports attached to their bodies. These survivors were very quiet, then someone new would walk in and the conversations about journeys would begin. These survivors were upbeat and determined, not a single hint of "poor me" from anyone. These survivors in their infirmity gave me hope.

The first look at my future was unsettling, yet strangely comforting. The wait with the ghost of my future was not very long though, and the next specter to appear was the reality of my present. A nurse with a medical record stood in the waiting room door, not unlike all the others on this journey.

"Janet Smith?"

Focus shifted to the sound of my name, away from the information I so wanted to eavesdrop upon.

"Yes, I'm here." I stood and approached her. I did not look back at my future.

"Follow me, please."

We entered a room just around the corner.

"You are here for an information visit, is that correct?"

"Yes, with Dr. Steve Wolff," answering back, rather meekly and atypically submissive.

"Have a seat. Dr. Wolff will be right with you."

With no fanfare or further word she left the room. The door slowly closed, leaving me in that box, waiting for the next man who would alter my life. As was my obsession, I began observing my environment.

There was the typical clinic exam room again, somewhat more used than the ones at Baptist: green paint, padded table, desk empty of anything but outdated magazines, and a few chairs positioned around the floor. Seems there was nothing new here.

Reading was the new distraction as time had to be filled while waiting for a doctor. I don't remember what it was, something by Spong, I think. Before the first sentence was read the door popped open. Startled, I looked up to see a tall, thin, dark-headed man (a cyclist, I would learn) breeze into the room with such energy I almost laughed. Tracy Dobbs was right, he was a little hyper. This very direct, smiling man in a white coat sat in a chair opposite me while his student sat next to me. He stuck out his hand in greeting.

Hello! Steve Wolff."

He introduced the student who was under his tutelage that month. We shook hands. It had been her job to find the newest information on my disease.

"I understand you are here seeking information, so how can I help you to understand what's ahead?"

Wolff took the bull by the horns. Good characteristic in my book. Wolff was very frank; another good quality, in my view. I've never known him to mince words since that first meeting.

"Janet, we looked at the biopsy slides Dr. Dobbs sent to us. The cells were somewhat crushed but they were such that we could make a diagnosis and we agree with Dr. Dobbs."

No real surprises, and I don't remember saying much. There were questions asked that were important to have answers to at this moment of the journey. He continued with the medical discussion.

"Janet, AMM, agnogenic myeloid metaplasia, causes scar tissue in the marrow. It starts as an altered stem cell becomes more responsive to growth factors whose activities become amplified. We don't know why. Some people have a chromosome change; we will test you for that change. I have given you a paper on the test and the factor. It is referred to as the Philadelphia chromosome."

"Could the cause have been an environmental exposure?" I asked, thinking back over my life experience as a chemist.

"It's possible; we will probably never know. It really doesn't matter. That is not our focus here."

I recoiled as he said it didn't matter. Sure, it mattered to me and my family, anyway.

Deep down though, I knew that was a true statement. Knowing how the disease was contracted would not change the fact, nor change the way my doctor would treat the disease. Dr. Wolff offered medical journal articles, and reiterated the terminal nature of AMM.

Janet, AMM is a slow mover. You have probably been ill for at least 10 or 15 years. At this moment in time, you are still fairly stable, although you have a few factors that make your prognosis a little less positive. Well, you need to see if you have a match. If you don't find a family match, you will go on the National Marrow Donor list. We will start with your siblings. Did you fill out the form we sent you?"

Gee whiz, those donor forms, again!

"No, I didn't, I want to talk to other people before I jumpstart this show."

"That's fine, but don't wait too long. You need to find a donor. If you don't have one in your family it can take a while."

Wolff was winding up. That phrase "take a while" was all I heard. And the time frame 10 to 15 years: that was around the time I had pneumonia, wasn't it?

Dr. Wolff said he was going to present my case at rounds the next day. To be sure, my rare case of AMM was brought up many times after that first session. The docs discuss all of the cases as to status and expected movement toward transplant. Multitudes of decisions were to be made and the transplant team would decide how medically prudent the choices would be at that moment. What a wonderful, informative, respectful, knowledgeable and egoless doctor you were, Steven Wolff, thank you.

I came home and called the siblings. The consensus was to talk to others before making a decision as to where I would have my transplant. Larry had been talking with other people in the medical field. He had easy access and he recommended Joseph Antin at Dana-Farber in Boston, Wolff had recommend Nelson Choa at Duke, and mentioned the Fred Hutchison Center in Seattle, the nation's premier hospital for transplant medicine. My sister Becky had a working relationship with someone whose brother worked for the NIH. Over the next month there was opportunity to speak with or visit with each of these sources.

All gave me the same answer: a rare disease, don't know much about it. Only a handful of people have looked at it at all. The litany of what was known was imprinted on my brain by now. The doctor would start the talk and my brain would finish it in textbook form.

Myelofibrosis affects about 3,000 people a year, mostly people over 60, and thus is seen as a normal result of an aging marrow. This group generally will die of something else entirely because the rate of change is so slow.

AMM, as a disease process, is found in a population of about 0.5 to 1.5 people per 100,000 persons tested. Only 22 percent of patients are under 56 years, 11 percent under 46 years of age (I had been having symptoms, which I ignored, for at least seven years by this time). The cause in this younger group is most often unknown. It is suspected that environmental exposure could induce the DNA change.

This DNA change alters the growth factor (a chemical in our body which turns on cell division and growth) responsiveness of the stem cell line making fibrocytes, a cell line responsible for healing and structure. The fibrocyte stem cell line proliferates at an unchecked rate, never stopping the production of fibrocytes, and eventually these cells fill all the space in the bone cavity, thus the term myelo (marrow)-fibrosis (scarring). Immature marrow cells of both red and white varieties are pushed out of the marrow cavity and into the bloodstream too quickly because there is no room to mature in the scarring cavity; thus the term a myeloproliferative disease.

With time, the red cell line decreases in number and because the red cell contains our hemoglobin that value also decreases and by definition anemia develops. The white cell lines, which consist of neutrophils, lymphocytes, etc., increase in number peripherally. Platelets, which are involved in our ability to clot, increase in the peripheral blood. Releasing them as immature cells they are expected to do the work they were assigned to do, as if they were fully mature. They cannot fill the bill.

Thankfully, our body is nothing if not redundant. A true blessing for anyone, ill or not, as it will find a way to work until it cannot do the work anymore.

Welcome our secondary hematopoetic (blood forming) sites to the world of AMM, my body's struggling knight in shining armor. The spleen, normally a blood repository organ and secondary site for making blood cells, tries to both clean up the abnormal circulating cells so rudely kicked out of their home and attempts making normal marrow cells.

Eventually, it too becomes so affected it has to enlarge. That can lead to liver complications if left too long, because of the increasing blood volume into the liver from a spleen that is holding more blood than is normal. The liver will also try to help with cleaning and repairing the blood so it enlarges.

A series of overloaded sponges being fed by garden hoses develops, if you will. In time, the heart has to work harder to deal with all of the blood behind it carried in these huge overworked organs.

A cascading series of events unfolds that will result in death if not checked. Dr. Mindell had been quite correct in his notation of a disease. The logical progression of this disease was frighteningly obvious.

The median survival time of patients after diagnosis is about three to six years. Benzene and toluene have been shown a causal link in some studies. Other than that, they did not know much about the cause. The only cure known was a stem cell transplant. With that, a 65 percent chance of a cure and a 33 percent chance of failure: read that as death or severe graft versus host disease.

There has been some new talk of a different prepping treatment called a mini-transplant; they'll see if it is appropriate.

Not too bad for a life and death struggle. While logical, it still seemed like the proverbial pig in the poke. Don't quite know what you are buying.

Trust, Janet.

CHAPTER EIGHTEEN

"Reach out and touch someone."

After Becky found out about my disease she started looking for information to help me and the family. She found the Leukemia Society and the bone marrow registry. She e-mailed every doctor she could find that would give her information. Becky was shocked and thrilled at the response she received from the doctors she had e-mailed. She gave donations to the Bone Marrow Donor Registry and recommended I talk with other people with my disease.

Those people turned out to be few and far between, as the statistics indicated. A total of five contacts were made during this time. The problem with this was that this was Becky's suggestion for approach, not mine. It filled her agenda for answers, but was not what I needed.

My need was to go on this journey with no preconceived ideas. I tried to remind Sis of this in terms of her own choice, not to hear others' stories of tonsillectomies before she had her surgery. Journeys like this needed only medical, logical, helpful information to make choices. Other's journeys could bog down the process. I had a hard enough time keeping my own fears out of the way. I knew I had no room for, or emotional stamina to deal with, theirs too at this moment.

Myelofibrosis was in charge of the path of this process but I had control over how I handled its effect on my approach methods along that path. As Proust had written, this was a journey only I could take; others may travel into and out of the journey, but the trip was mine and I had to make it mine.

A few people with the disease or family members of people with the disease contacted me by e-mail. Some had survived their transplant: good news for my family. Most were on disability, looking for options other than transplant. In my arrogance, generated from my need of being a lone ranger in this, I felt they were afraid to go for the cure and it translated to me as a fear of death.

Undoubtedly, this was a harsh judgment made without facts, and thus I apologize to them for my temporary inability to sustain thoughts of someone else's plight. For this traveler, an emotional approach was not the kind of approach I understood. Their trial, no matter how valid, how painful, how honest, how hopeless, was not my experience.

People handle their travels based on their own life knowledge. My life knowledge was too narrow around this issue and I could not relate to the place they were coming from in that moment. Maybe they had just learned of their disease, maybe they had a family for whom they feared; I do not know. But, even now, I am wont to compare illnesses in people. Each of us has his own path to follow. These paths are not comparable in origin or effect. What is easy for one will be absolutely devastating to another. I choose not to deal in comparisons.

Having said that, I appreciated them, felt for them, but at this moment in my life could not focus on their needs for communication and fretting over their future. Bigger fish needed frying. A selfish need to focus on myself and my family and my own resolve in dealing with this event reared its ugly head. This resolve admonished me: move on and make choices based on my read of the information, given to me by my doctors of my situation in any given moment.

The process demanded of me that I let go and let God. As a result of that letting go I had to have the faith to trust my doctors and the choices we made together. My family became a cocoon and they gave freely the love, time and space I needed to prepare for this ultimate life choice, the consequences of which would literally mean life or death.

By now, my church knew and the churches of my family and friends knew of my illness. They were there and are still there, rocks of faith, all. God Bless them! The prayers were to be lifted up from across the nation in ways I never thought possible. God's grace was present. My wisdom was growing.

CHAPTER NINETEEN

"Yet oh, why should they know their fate,
Since sorrow never comes too late,
And happiness too swiftly flies?

Thought would destroy their paradise,
No more, where ignorance is bliss,
'Tis folly to be wise."

Thomas Gray

After choosing Vanderbilt as my transplant center, Dr. Wolff needed to run more tests. He did not have to reconfirm the diagnosis but all doctors redo older tests and add new ones. The doctor-patient relationship is established and they define the problem by their institution's parameters and develop baselines for future reference. It keeps everyone honest.

The testing began by having many tubes of my blood filled for multiple DNA, viral and bacterial testing. A brief list might include HLA typing, or human leukocyte antigen typing, which gives the doctor the best information to determine the donor; blood typing and matching; cytomegalo virus (CMV) titer; hepatitis titers; herpes virus; HIV/AIDS; toxoplasmosis; tuberculosis; and on and on and on.

A patient has a better chance to survive a transplant if they are negative for all of these pathogens, but just because you have a positive reaction to some of the tests, does not mean a "no go" for the transplant. The adage "forewarned is forearmed" is the by word in this case.

Myself, I had a positive CMV titer. I was surprised, that as a veterinarian, a fan of gardening and eating a nice slice of medium rare prime rib from time to time, that I did not have a positive toxoplasmosis titer. I was lucky to be negative. Finding a donor with 6/6 HLA sites was imperative now. To digress a little I will try to relate what HLA is about.

So that our body can protect itself from disease, it has the ability to recognize invading organisms or cells. It constantly asks itself, "Is this or is this not me?"

To aid this chore humans have a gland called the thymus located in our chest, which reduces in size and function over time. It is one of the responsibilities of this gland to teach our body what "self" is so the immune system will know "not self." To do this, the thymus gland marks certain lymphocytes that were bathed in its environment with the ability to recognize our body tissues as "self". These T-cells (thymus-cells) are one of our body's police force members, along with B-cells (Bursa-cells) and other killer cells and cell released toxins found in our white blood cell line.

Our T-cells and B-cells continuously cruise our blood vessels and tissues searching for and recognizing the abnormal markers on cells or organisms in our body as either "self" or "not self." When a foreign organism, "not self", enters our body they respond by a calling to arms our body defense system. Our white blood cells then attack the intruding body, or the antigen-antibody complex activates, or both (cellular immunity or humoral immunity). An easy reference is an allergen, or a delayed hypersensitivy reaction like poison ivy, or flu or bacteria or our own tissues as in an autoimmune disease, or antibodies built up due to vaccinations; whatever the invader an attack will occur.

In the case of transplant, if you have a donor with the same HLA sites (which are simply surface protein markers our cells expose to the world) as the recipient, then the chance for "self-recognition" becomes amplified and our immune system more easily accepts the "foreign" cell type of the donor as equal to that of the recipient's body. If one is not so lucky to find this match then the unmatched cell sites give the donor/recipient T-cells opportunity to go on the defensive/offensive against the transplant patient.

This reaction of donor cells to recipient, or vice-versa, is the basis for graft vs. host disease or the opposite of that, rejection of the graft. Some reaction is needed but it must stay under control. The typing test looks for six of the major antigens or proteins located on the cell surface. Know there are many more minor surface antigens, but a 6/6 major loci find is considered a perfect match.

Most often, a family member will match, though I had heard stories of people who had multiple siblings and could not find a sibling match. None of the other siblings matched anyone in the family of 10! Surely, one of my brothers or one of my sisters would match so that I would not have to enter the marrow donor system.

I had four options, many more than most, hopefully enough. DNA recombination during embryo formation has many possibilities. I had to believe I was not to be left out in the cold without a match; no pun intended. This disease had been hanging around for at least ten or fifteen years. I had known something was not right but fortunately lived without the definitive knowledge; what a blessing. Gray was right. Ignorance can be bliss.

Now I knew and the consequences of this disease would no longer allow ignorance as an excuse for not being present for my life. Action, great doctors and faith were all I had, outside of my family's and my friends' unstoppable support.

During this time of definition it became apparent that the patient was not the only entity involved in the process of transplant medicine. Laura had to have an aide at Andrews pull her blood for the HLA and disease tests and mail them to Vandy; she could not get time away to come to Tennessee. Becky had her blood pulled in Atlanta and sent to Vanderbilt. My cousin Mary offered to be tested. The doctors felt that if none of my siblings matched she could be tested. They waited because the testing is expensive and is usually at the patient's full cost.

While my brothers were at Vandy having their blood tested for disease and HLA typing, they stepped into a room with one of the doctors and discussed finances around the transplant. How is this going to be paid for, how much will insurance cover? They were able to take the initial inquiry about costs off my plate. My brothers did not fill me in on what they had learned. They too felt I had enough to deal with and did not need to know. I could not alter the business end of what was to come. This was in July and August of 2000. The donor search was on and it was a very specific requirement, one often difficult to meet.

Laura was farther away than any of my siblings, as she was stationed in Maryland at Andrews Air Force Base. She felt she had nothing to offer. In my heart I knew better. She was Neldie, and I knew she would not be a silent factor in the game.

My younger sister Becky is a doer of the first order. She was, and continues to be, my advocate. She organized the entire outside show. Transplants create a need to form a new world for the family and the patient to live in during and after the process. She placed me on prayer lists across the country. She took care of the worldly problems. She started developing the logistical plan that would carry us through the next two years, leaving me in a position to be able to focus on my body's needs and my soul's preparation in case of death. That search for a path through to the other side of disease would be an all-encompassing pursuit and one that needed to be my only focus at this stage. There was nothing else I could do.

CHAPTER TWENTY

"Really? Who is it?"

Still working 35-40 hours a week, days were becoming more and more difficult but I was not going to give in to this disease so quickly. The job kept my mind from wandering and a room full of puppies was just the medicine needed. Solving another sentient creature's problems gave me hope my doctors would solve mine.

Time gave my illness permission to become obvious and all the staff knew how sick I was, what I was facing, and the resultant possibility of death. Their support was touching. One of the technicians' fiancé was suffering from a marrow disease and was going to Vandy. He had already had his typing done for a transplant and to date has not needed the procedure.

Weeks had passed since the HLA testing and I was feeling a good deal of stress about the results of the search. Walking in to the break room of the clinic to have lunch, I decided to call Dr. Wolff.

His voice came on the line,

"Steve Wolff, how can I help you?"

"Dr. Wolff, this is Janet Smith, how are you?"

"Doing great, what do you need?" always to the point.

"I was wondering if you had gotten any of the antigen typing results back."

That little bearer of fear was sitting on my shoulder whispering the greatest fear of all; what if I had no match?

"I don't know, haven't seen them, let me look." There was a pause as he checked the computer.

"Janet, nothing yet. I'll let you know soon as I do."

"Thanks Steve, talk to you later." I hung up.

Everyone there that day was as disappointed as I. Taking my sandwich out of my lunch sack I started to take a bite. Too nervous to eat I closed the bag, drank my bottled water and chatted with the staff.

Three minutes later, the phone rang. I just grabbed it, unusual; doctors usually don't answer the clinic phone.

"Hello?"

I heard Steve's voice, "May I speak with Dr. Janet?"

"This is she."

My heart began to pound, the silence seemed a lifetime.

Dr. Steve joyfully belted out, "Laura Rodriguez!"

My heart leapt! I was dancing in place, Becky's happy dance, and tears of joy were streaming down my cheeks.

"I knew it! I knew Nell would be the one! Thanks, Steve, I've got to call Laura."

The excitement was overwhelming. I had a match. My match was the one who thought they would have no role. I could not wait to tell Neldie!

"Talk to you later, Janet, glad you got a match." Steve hung up.

All of my siblings had a role; Laura's became the life-saving role. Relieved I had a 6/6 match I relaxed, knowing there was an option.

Right now, I had to call Laura. I picked up the phone and dialed Andrews Air Force Base. The phone began to ring.

"Major Rodriguez, how may I help?"

"Sis, I just talked with Dr. Wolff and we know who the donor is."

I was trying to be so contained.

"Really, who is it?"

"It's you Neldie, I knew it would be."

Silence dominated the other end of the line. Suddenly afraid, I wondered had I had assumed too much? Then I remembered this was Neldie, the girl who would give the shirt off her back to someone who needed it more than she. I was always watching her back when we were kids, waiting for someone to take advantage of her good nature.

"Laura, are you okay?"

"Yes, I'm fine." I could hear the tears in her voice.

"I'm glad it's me; glad I can help, Sis. I love you."

"I love you too, Neldie. Thank you, talk soon, bye."

Again, I had only tears of joy in the thought a path out of the forest had suddenly become so clear. Laura sold her motorcycle, a dream of hers for years. She said it could keep a while longer.

Over the next few days all of the results came in and I found that both of my brothers matched me 6/6 as well, another blessing for my life. Larry said he wished he could have been my donor, but was happy it was Laura, his "twinlet." The down side, Becky only matched by three or four antigens. My heart broke, praying she would never need a transplant. Her attitude was, well, I just have other work to do around this. I'll be fine.

Now, Laura, being property of the United States government, had to seek permission to be my donor. She filed papers with AFMOA, and sought permission from the medical consultants. The government said she could be my donor but they would not accept any responsibility for testing or any consequence of being my donor, financial or medical or career-wise, if something occurred that made her unemployable in the USAF.

Since it was a case of life or death her commanding officers at Andrews approved the time away she would need to be my donor. This was July 2000, three short months since diagnosis. A true miracle occurred when her availability for the transplant was approved so early.

CHAPTER TWENTY-ONE

"Some folks' lives roll easy, some folks' lives never roll at all, they just fall, ooooh they just fall…"

Paul Simon

Believe me, I am not complaining or looking for sympathy when I say my life has traditionally been one of struggle; people do struggle so I am not special in that experience. I own being the cause of a lot of that strife from poor choices and self-inflicted damage.

Paul Simon's song, "Some Folks' Lives" seemed to almost be an anthem. It seemed every time I thought I was heading down the right path some event would occur that destroyed that illusion, or taught me a lesson I should not have had to learn through experience. One of my dad's favorite adages was, "Janet, you don't have to experience everything to understand it; learn from others choices."

Took me a while and a few 2 x 4's but I got that one.

Ultimately those struggles made me stronger and the trials became my gifts. Labeled as Mom's sensitive child and I own that, I did and still sometimes do get emotional, empathetic, sympathetic, even angry and vocal over issues and situations that fill life. I suppose my life to point was prepping me for the most difficult fight I would ever face, and the ordeals I forged through made me stronger, made me more able to sift through the emotionalism quickly and get to the core of the issue facing me at the moment.

Even though I sometimes wondered what would happen next, I knew in my soul I would muddle through and come out stronger. I always had, why would it change now? Never mind the fact I had a tremendous role model in my Dad. What a wonderful example to follow in how to deal with adversity in your daily life.

A diabetic with cardiovascular disease and diabetic neuropathies, Dad lived his life with gusto and very much in the moment. Even though mostly blind from bilateral retinal detachments, and mostly deaf from all those years of flying, he would still work at the agency every day and go to his garage every evening and work on some piece of equipment or his boat motor. He could not see to place a bolt but he knew where it should go and he could feel to place it. He knew engines so well he could tell when he had it right.

He was devoted to his family and he loved living his life, always doing what he had loved. He helped people every day, changing lives. He wanted everyone to reach their maximum abilities. He pushed others the way he did his kids: go, be, and try. He never complained about his health, no matter how many times I asked, "Pa, ya feeling OK this morning?" His answer was always yes and he was always laughing and smiling. I wish he had complained more; he might still be with us.

As strong as Dad was in his own battle, he would have had a very difficult time seeing me go through what I was going to have to endure. The consequences of my ultimate choice would have terrified him. Dad was a fretter when it came to his children. He was a fixer and this would have been out of his range of repair talents.

Nevertheless, Dad gave me a road map for the fight in how he led his life. The faith in God's grace that led me to my soul's resolve to face this event daily, with faith in a positive outcome, would have been more difficult to rely on had I not seen my father handle his bumps in the road. Dad and Mother also raised their children to be there for their siblings. Dad fixed things for me quite nicely.

The knowledge that all of the events I was experiencing would eventually come to a good end (regardless of that end), kept me moving through the journey. I focused on my dad often during my experience, trying to remember his voice and his attitude and his words of love. I was determined to face this disease head on.

Even with my bravada, I was having a very hard time seeing myself on the other side of this disease. The future had no light; at this moment it was all amorphous gray and obscured. Not knowing how to regain that light was forcing me into a different view of what life I had left in this world. I resigned myself to the path chosen for my future and focused on preparing for my death. Thinking I could now move forward in dealing with this threat to my life, another event would intervene and shake this tenuous security in the future a bit further. I really was not ready for what was next.

CHAPTER TWENTY-TWO

"Riverglen and the gift of David"

One weekend in of the middle of August 2000, the weather was horrible, pouring rain. Of course it would be; there was a three-day horse trial at Riverglen Farm in New Market, Tennessee. Traci was riding her new horse. A couple of other friends of Traci's and peripherally mine, David, who also had Steve for a physician, and his companion Elaine, were attending the event.

I had last seen David at Traci's wedding in '92, and I had kept up with David and his struggle through Traci. I had seen Elaine at the Rolex earlier in the year at the Kentucky Horse Park. David was there, but was out riding his bike through the Kentucky horse farm region. "Happy as a clam" was how Elaine described David on his bike.

By the time the cross-country phase had begun at Riverglen, the weather had cleared and those hills had become East Tennessee muggy and southern August hot. Mist began rising from the ground and collected in the lower areas where the hills met. Our rain-soaked clothes were starting to stick to our skin as we climbed one of the hills to get a view of the course.

Elaine, David and I caught each other up on our lives as we watched the other riders take their turns. We were near the water complex. Traci's horse in the past had not wanted to hit the water. Her new horse could care less and was bent on finishing the course in rapid time. We had to get cameras ready if we wanted to catch a good shot over a jump. I sat down next to David. He admitted he would have much rather been off somewhere on his bike, but he was gracious in his loss of that indulgence for the day.

As we waited for Traci to approach the nearest jump, David and I chatted about how we were feeling. An avid cyclist, David was regularly riding and even though he looked strong, he still had a pale countenance and his hair seemed to have never grown back in evenly.

David had had lymphoma and had endured two transplants, one auto (self donor) and one allo (foreign donor). David was one brave, determined, sweet guy. He had had many GVHD problems and was on immunosuppressants for a long time. I had so much respect for David and how he had handled his journey. I was fearful of going through the long hell David had had to experience. In the trials of David, God gave me another example to reflect upon during my passage toward health or death.

While sitting on the wet ground getting our cameras ready, David turned his head in my direction and quietly asked, "Did you know Steve is considering leaving Vanderbilt and doing only research?"

He kept looking at me, waiting for a reaction; then he quickly dropped his head. Looking at the ground and picking at the grass he almost visibly seemed to regret what had just left his lips.

"Is he really?" Think ambivalence, Janet. "Do you really think he will leave?"

The fear of Steve's leaving was in my voice, I heard it.

David dropped his head a little more and then looked back up at me, knowing what I would lose should Steve leave Vanderbilt.

"Yeah, I do. I think he's ready for a change."

The conversation ended as Traci came through the water and headed for a vertical jump with a ditch on the other side. I aimed my camera and nothing! It froze. Just great, oh, well.

I let the information David had given me slide, but I did not forget. I trusted Steve from the moment I had met him. His honest demeanor and rich base of knowledge and experience with transplant medicine was reassuring. His character was obvious. Steve was a good man and a fantastic doctor. I was hoping David was wrong.

After Traci's run of the course, I said my goodbyes and left the farm. I never saw David again. The following February, David was diagnosed with squamous cell carcinoma in his esophagus. He was to undergo surgical removal of the mass that same month. If he survived, he may never be able to speak again. He was really frightened this time, sure the reaper had his ticket.

A specialist, accustomed to performing this type of surgery, was flown in to remove the mass. David made it through surgery, but he developed a bleed during the night while in ICU. David bled to death before the surgeons could stop the loss. David died the day after Valentine's Day, 2001.

Elaine is still devastated by this loss, an unexpected end to the many years of struggle, and has not yet recovered from the suddenness of David's death. The good news: Elaine and I, over time, have forged a friendship through the pain of this common experience. Elaine is focusing on her future now, getting much stronger and moving forward in her life.

CHAPTER TWENTY-THREE

"Our own physical body possesses a wisdom which we who inhabit the body lack."

Henry Miller

The days toward the end of the year 2000 became more difficult physically. Time for a choice and with that choice would come the obligatory consequence.

Mentally and, more importantly, spiritually I had finally come to a position of peace. My prayers and meditations and acceptance of the facts of my present had brought moments where there was comfort with what was ahead. Not to be fooled, I was still having difficulty envisioning life on the other side of this disease. The new reality was that I was learning to be comfortable with the concept of dying if that was to be my fate.

Life had brought many deaths to our family and the realization that life continues without the one who has passed really hit home. Learning to remove my fear of thoughts of the future of my family without me in it began to be easy. They would manage quite well.

What was left was my need to fully let go of all sentiments and things the world contained. New perspectives were forming around my concept of this life.

My spirit blessed my mind and body with a unique method to pull away from the rigors of this life and death journey I had embarked upon. "I" seemed to be separating from my body. There came a quiet realization that my spirit was not ill at all, only my physical body was ill. "I" cared about my body, but there was a benign detachment. This detachment allowed me to make emotionless choices concerning my treatment and my future or lack of one.

Whatever "I" was experiencing, the reality of that knowledge came to be my salvation through the days ahead. Even so, there were still many unanswered questions and a definite level of fear of the unknown. My first fear had to be approached; the moment had come for my first major decision. What will come when I get rid of this "alien spleen" inside of me? "Spleen baby" had to be "born."

My ability to eat had dropped precipitously because of the pain a full stomach caused. Eating many very small meals daily did not make any difference; it still hurt. G.I. function was abnormal, shifting from constipation to diarrhea and always bloated. Exhaustion was a constant companion. Dr. Dobbs and I discussed the possibility of surgery.

My first appointment was with a surgeon in Knoxville. He said he had never removed a spleen as large as mine but was confident he would do a good job. It was not that I did not trust the surgeon. I wanted to talk to someone else before making my decision. Dr. Dobbs called Vanderbilt and got a recommendation from Dr. Wolff. I really wanted to have history there before the transplant. I also knew Vanderbilt would have a surgeon around that had seen and removed a spleen as enlarged as mine.

In March 2001, I had an appointment to see Dr. William C. Chapman, a surgeon whose group would ultimately be responsible for removing my spleen. I entered the exam room and was only by myself a few moments. The door opened and a medium-height, dark-headed laughing man entered the room.

"Janet, Dr. Chapman, let's talk about why you want your spleen out now."

Straight up, I can deal with that attitude. Dr. Chapman was a pleasant man, very calm, and a good listener, and he had a history with horses. He had to have the right stuff, all good characteristics to have in a surgeon. A liver transplant specialist, "hemostasis" was his middle name. Knowing how to control blood loss is a very important skill when you remove a spleen like mine.

"Doctor Chapman, I am miserable. I can't eat, I can't get comfortable, I am exhausted, and honestly, I don't want to be extremely ill before we remove my spleen. Why wait until my liver is involved or my disease worsens?"

I looked at him as directly as I could and felt I had made my case with a good amount of logic. I kept asking, "Is it not better to go into the transplant feeling more well than not well?"

Dr. Chapman nodded his head.

"Janet, I do agree with the majority of those reasons. The main one for not taking it out right now is the likelihood your transplant might not be far behind. You could stay stable for a while after the spleen is removed, but you might not. We just don't want to put you at great risk unnecessarily."

He was right, but my years of being a veterinarian taught me there is much to be said for "quality" of life.

"I appreciate that, Dr. Chapman, but I am 'over' this spleen. I want it gone."

Chapman said he needed to call Steve. He stepped out of the room to call, but not before sending in a medical student.

"Janet, do you mind if my student palpates your spleen? We do not often get a patient with a spleen we can feel."

The student walked in with an uncertain look on her face. I am sure she did not want me to feel like a guinea pig.

"Sure, that's fine." Chapman walked out the door.

The student walked in the exam room and closed the door. Having been a veterinary student, I knew these kinds of opportunities were golden. I was soon thinking that she did not find this an opportunity, period. Her exam was very tentative, disinterested even. I encouraged her to find the extent of the spleen's place in my abdomen. She meekly palpated the spleen margins and left, and left me with the impression her interests were not in surgery or oncology.

Chapman spoke with Wolff about his exam and our discussion, the choice made, the consequences of that choice defined. Chapman's orders were to go to the Hillsboro imaging center and have an abdominal CT before leaving Nashville. The Vanderbilt radiology department was packed.

The lab gave me two bottles of opaque media so the spleen would stand out on the film. Procedure was to drink a bottle every 30 minutes, one on my way down the street to the center and the other while sitting in the parking lot waiting for the appointment time. Bloated with contrast, I entered the CT room and the technician walked in behind me.

"Janet, did you drink the contrast?"

"Yes."

"Then go ahead and lie down on the table, feet first. I will ask you to hold your breath from time to time during this scan. It will take about 20 minutes."

Same procedure as at Baptist almost a year ago; the tech was right—20 minutes later and I was out of there, heading back down I-40 east and home. I don't remember the ride, but felt completely at ease with what had been discussed with Dr. Chapman, with his team's abilities to remove my grossly enlarged spleen, and with the consequences of the removal.

CHAPTER TWENTY-FOUR

"A change in the guard"

There had been no news from Chapman or Wolff since my appointment on March 7 and it was nearing the end of the month. I sent an e-mail to Steve asking about the decision around the surgery. The message back indicated the transplant team had agreed the surgery was a good choice at this moment. Dr. Chapman would set the date and his office would contact me with the exact date and time to come back for the pre-op testing.

Hidden at the end of his response was a statement that really sent me for a loop. David had been right; Steve was leaving Vanderbilt at the end of the month and going into research in the private sector.

He said that he was sorry if his decision was going to cause any upset; that he realized a doctor-patient relationship was established and he hoped I could find another relationship that would work well.

As my heart sank, and my stomach turned, the only way I could describe my emotions were shock, then anger and finally a sense of betrayal. All of these feelings pounded my body within milliseconds of each other; I was thrown into a mini-state of shock. My bond had already developed with him as my doctor. David had depended on him, teaching me that I could too. I trusted Dr. Wolff. My future was in his hands. Suddenly, and almost without warning, he was giving it back to me at that moment and in an informal e-mail.

A reactionary missile launched toward Wolff. What was I going to do? Now I had to find a new doctor, blah, blah, blah. I was not happy. I went offline, confused, frightened and unsure of what was next. Suddenly my life to point seemed based upon shifting sands and I had to get my feet back onto something level, something solid and fast.

After a few moments and a few deep breaths, I regained my composure and mailed Dr. Wolff back. I apologized for reacting so incredulously, not really so sure I meant that apology. He could have called me and told me by voice, at least. However, that did not happen. The thought of my having to leave Vanderbilt and of having to go out of state for this transplant was not in my plan book. Reaching this conclusion left me only one choice.

I asked Dr. Wolff who he would feel comfortable referring me to within his transplant team at Vanderbilt. His response was multifold, but one doctor stood out in description. His name was Dr. Madan Jagasia. Wolff described him as a young doctor on the staff. He and his wife were both on staff. He was pictured as very bright and a fighter, an excellent doctor. Steve was transferring many of his cases to Dr. Madan. I said, "OK."

I am grateful that I made the choice to stay within the Vanderbilt group, grateful Dr. Wolff referred my case into Dr. Madan's care and I am grateful Dr. Steve remained in my loop. His experience and knowledge of transplant medicine was a gift I did not want to lose. Steve's second gift to me was Madan. When you commit your life into someone else's hands, you need to know they are going to be there. Dr. Madan Jagasia took over my case when Wolff left Vanderbilt at the end of March 2001, and he has been there ever since.

Madan is tall, dark-haired, dark-eyed, handsome, affable, calm, an extremely capable and intelligent man. Since the time Dr. Jagasia took over my case, he has been a rock. He is always a great source of medical knowledge, as egoless as Steve, and a great listener. He is willing to be a friend when needed, a drill sergeant when needed, a huge reality check when needed, the light at the end of my tunnel when things were not quite right, and overall a wonderful doctor, and human being.

Before my splenectomy, I had my first appointment with Dr. J. Mom drove up with me for that visit. As Madan walked us through the surgery consequences, the subsequent transplant, and the consequences of that choice, I noticed my mom's wise blue eyes tear up. I have only seen my mother cry two or three times in my life. This was the first time I had seen her cry over my dilemma. It was heart-wrenching for me. She turned her face toward Dr. Jagasia and in a few choice words all of her fears were placed on the table.

"I just want her to live. Please do what you have to do."

Dr. J. dropped his head for a moment and said he would do all he could to make that happen.

A mother should never have to bury a child of any age; it happens all too often in this world. I became determined to not have my mother experience that grief.

I vividly remember that day and that room. The paint was a dull gray-green on a wall constructed of sheet rock with greenish paint and paper. The floor was typical hospital linoleum. The door was a dark metal gray. A desk was against the wall to the left of the door. An exam table was placed into the corner extending into the middle of the room. A sink and cabinet were against the right wall. A curtain could separate the room into two parts. Fluorescent lighting filled the room. It was cold.

Sitting on a gray vinyl-covered metal chair between Mom and Dr. J., I felt like I was in a vacuum tube, very cold to my core and slowly running out of air to breathe. I zoned away from the noise and the reality for a moment and sensed that the air in my vacuum tube continued to be removed. I was suffocating under the weight of the pressure that my truth was creating. Their voices slowly muted. My body was present, I heard the conversations, understood the medicine, and fully appreciated what my life would bring in the immediate future. I was so tired of all the words, all the running back and forth, all the waiting for results, all the fear, all the unknown factors. My future became a wearing thought that day.

With this visit I realized that I had officially become my disease. Janet Smith DVM now had AMM stamped on her forehead, scarlet letters for the world to see.

Looking much further into the future than that moment, though, reminded me that I was still having a very difficult time seeing myself on the other side of the disease. No matter how I tried to move forward the same question kept coming into my mind. How do you move past something that is as inherently defining as a terminal disease? Looking much farther did not profit me at all; I finally accepted my life had become a life measured only in moments. That would have to be enough time to finish my business here in this life.

This may sound trite, clichéd, whatever your term for the obvious, but I believe we react to life-and-death situations in this way because it is a truth. Life becomes a one-day deal. Until that moment of recognition and acceptance that our own mortality has thrust itself upon our consciousness, we do not fully comprehend how our life is really only measured in the moments we live. Life is not in the possibility of moments to come our way. Moments are the only life we have.

However, belief in moments to come gives us hope. Those future moments sustain the will to live and fight. Hope is the essential motivator. I have never given up hope for my life. I admit getting crossways about some events, and I own the tangents. I still have hope.

After the appointment with Madan was finished, I was to go to the Red Cross office across the street from the Vanderbilt Clinic. They removed a pint of blood for cross-matching and blood-typing and to have a replacement in case the surgeons needed blood during my splenectomy.

Mom and I returned home late that evening. We were exhausted. The day had taken its toll on Mother; I did not let her go back to Vanderbilt with me again. I traveled alone for my appointments. The process I had entered was so much easier to deal with alone, less explaining. I could control the flow of information to others that way. What they don't know won't hurt them.

CHAPTER TWENTY-FIVE

> "It is the power of the Other which pulls him upward out of his attachments to body and earth, cajoling him to do what he cannot do of himself...let go. This power, when so felt, we call grace. Let grace in by responding positively to the teaching and by letting go of the ego."
>
> Paul Bruton

By April 2001, my body was at the command of my disease and my doctors. I found myself grateful that I had had a few more moments than most to come to terms with this disease, the choices I would have to make, and my life to this point.

Grace gave to me the ability to so forgive myself for all those stupid things I had done in my life, and I had made plenty of stupid choices. Instead of becoming angry that this disease found me, I became grateful that the disease was an insidious, slow disease.

I became grateful that I had been ignorant of its existence for a long time. I had time, something many transplant patients don't have. My mind, or self, or soul, whatever you choose to call it, came to exist on another plane, transcending my body.

It was not an out-of-body experience like some describe. I was definitely present, but "I" was safe. God was giving me a safe harbor from the storm. He was allowing me an existence on earth apart from my body. He allowed me a way to objectively, and without emotion, deal with the choices that would need addressing during the journey. There was an enveloping peace; I had no fear of dying.

Having shed my fear of dying I became fully prepared to live. I prayed I would never lose this feeling of peace and acceptance. Maybe I was beginning to see life on the other side of AMM and a transplant. I had been blessed with not having to know for years, I had been blessed with excellent doctors, and I had been blessed with three family matches. I could see life, but that view was still hazy. Seeing me on the other side of this disease was going to be hard. If I was going to survive, I had to let go and find that view.

CHAPTER TWENTY-SIX

"Karma is the moral law of divine Being which is itself gracious. God's justice and God's mercy work together."

Geddes MacGregor

The splenectomy was scheduled for April 19, 2001. My friends had all called before I left for Vandy. Traci called and said she was going to visit Elaine and mentioned they would come to see me while I was recovering. I was stunned. Was she serious? I just kept wondering how Elaine would feel about that decision. So, old blunt me asked outright about that choice.

"Traci, don't you think the last place Elaine would want to be is Vanderbilt? It hasn't been much more than a month since losing David. I would love to see you both but why don't you just stay at Elaine's and not worry about visiting me?"

"I guess I didn't think about that, you're right. We will call you."

"Sure, fine. Tell Elaine hello and I am thinking of her."

"I will; bye." It was quite a while before I heard from her again.

My family all met in Nashville the night before the surgery. Jack treated us to early dinner at the Sunset Grill in Hillsboro Village and we drove back to our rooms to wait for the morning.

Morning presented itself as a cool, damp, dark day as we left the hotel to go to the hospital. Becky turned up the heat on the defroster. I had to be there around 6 a.m. I do not remember anything being said except, right, right, left, left, right, as we wandered towards Vandy and into the parking garage in front of the hospital.

Getting out of the car I froze as a slight wave of fear rode my spine and then disappeared into the fog of the morning. Taking a deep breath, a prayer was given that God would see me, my family and most importantly my medical team through this day. Grabbing my bag out of the trunk and making sure I had all of my legal papers, Becky and I walked across the street and into VUMC's lobby and waiting room. Jack brought Mom over a few moments behind. Larry and Laura were both flying in that morning and would not arrive until 10 a.m.

I sat down in the lobby and less than five minutes later my name was spoken out from across the room.

"Janet Smith?"

"Yes."

I looked up, turning toward the voice to the right of my chair. A dark-haired woman, dressed in a dark, suit was standing in the door of the admissions office.

"Will you step into admissions, please, and we will get you set up to go to pre-op."

"Here, have a seat and we will get this going. How are you doing?"

"Well, trying to not think about what is coming, trying to focus on my family."

"I understand; you will do fine."

I almost felt a separation from my body; I was watching the game begin from a most unusual seat. Janet was sitting there; "I" was an impassive observer of the scene. This must be one of those out-of-body deals, I kept thinking as she spoke.

"Do you have a living will on file here?"

"Yes, I have one but it is not yet on file."

"Did you bring it with you?"

"Yes."

"May I have it please?"

I handed the blue-backed legal paper to her.

"This will permanently be on file here now, whenever or if you need it again."

The notion that I was giving my doctors at Vanderbilt the right to ask my family permission to turn me off as we had done to my father was a chilling thought to deal with. I knew I did not want to just have bodily existence in this life and my choice was clear in that legal document. If I cannot contribute in this life, let me go. I do not want to exist in a disconnected, non-functioning body. I choose not to exist without an ability to cogitate and communicate; I do not want to exist with an inability to care for myself. No thanks. The emotional and financial costs of such a selfish choice were not going to be on my head. Let me go. Again, I believe in quality of life, not quantity. I had made that decision before seeing the lawyer and setting my position to paper.

The day I visited the lawyer to take care of my living will, medical power of attorney, and power of attorney was a bizarre time. Mr. Newcomb and Dad had been friends for years. Bill and I had a long chat about how much Dad had meant to him and that as a result he felt especially close to all of my family. We chatted about my disease and what I would have to undergo. Bill related his experience with cancer. He had been treated at Vanderbilt. We finished the business, Bill wished me best of luck, and sent his regards to Mother.

I was going home with two very important legal documents, one to cover death, and one to cover a bad outcome that would leave me hanging between life and death. I had already discussed with my family and had written down what I wanted in case of death.

With the exchange in the admissions office over, they called pre-op and said that I was ready. I took my seat in the lobby outside once again, holding my mother's hand and thankful for my sibling's love and support.

This surgery was risky. The chance for blood loss was great and the consequences of that loss were present in our minds. I was touched deeply by my siblings' presence, glad I could say goodbye before I went "under the knife." Mother did not say much, and hugged and kissed me with an "I love you. See you when it's done." Her faith and years of being a nurse overrode her fear.

At 7:30 a.m. on the 19th of April, one day before her birthday, Becky was next to me in pre-op. I had taken off all my clothes and put them in the little plastic bag. I had put on the ubiquitous hospital gown and the intravenous lines had been placed in my arm. I noticed the IV catheters were rather large-bore, reminding me that my engorged spleen could shatter like a watermelon on the pavement and start bleeding and how quickly the blood would pore into my abdominal cavity. Another vision I could have lived without at the moment.

Becky was smiling and laughing, talking to the nurse, engaging the morning's activities to help the time pass. She looked down at me and gave me what she thought was excellent news.

"Sis, there is good karma here today; your anesthesiologist is a woman."

I knew how hard it was for Becky, of all people, to be standing there with me in pre-op. She has always passed out when she thought too much about what someone she loved was experiencing. I really appreciated her presence. This was her way of thanking me for holding her hand the August before when she had her tonsils and adenoids removed and her sinuses scraped and her septum straightened. My anesthesiologist had ordered that her assistant give me an injection of Versed, a pre-anesthetic.

Within seconds, my body relaxed and my vision blurred.

A smiling anesthesiologist's face and the phrase, "There goes the wall," were my last visual and verbal memories of that morning.

The surgery was uneventful, I was told, in and out in an hour-and-a-half. My surgeons had blocked off and were expecting three to four hours surgery time. Fortunately, my spleen, not attached to other intestinal tissues, was easily accessible; it probably popped out of my abdomen like the "Alien spawn"!

Removal left me almost eight pounds lighter. The girls at the clinic had created a contest to see who could guess the correct weight of "Spleen Baby." Another gift given and received, an easy surgery, from the technical standpoint, anyway.

I startled awake around three or four in the afternoon to "There she is!" Larry and Laura were at my bedside. Mom and Jack were outside my room, as was Becky; she was slumped against the wall. She ran as soon as I made my first groan!

The pain was unbelievable, shaking uncontrollably with each movement or deep breath. Cut from my sternum to past my umbilicus my core muscles were damaged and I could not move without severe pain. The morphine pump seemed worthless at times, especially when I was too out of it to find the button, yet in it enough to know I needed to find that button.

My surgery team came in daily. Dr. Chapman came on the second day and seemed pleased with the results. He was standing at the foot of my bed with his surgical team when the bandage was removed.

"Subcuticular, huh?" he said to his chief resident.

With that, I felt he had probably watched his chief resident do the surgery and left after all had gone well. No matter, he had been there if things had gone afoul.

"Good job".

The resident beamed; all good deeds should be honored. I had asked for that type of skin closure before the surgery. I did not want a huge scar down the middle of my abdomen. Vanity, oh vanity, all is vanity; guess reality does sneak into life-and-death situations, always hope! The surgeon did do a good job; the scar is only pencil-lead wide.

Later in the afternoon of the second day a few of the hem/onc doctors came by to say hello to their new AMM patient. Dr. Stein introduced himself and said he had heard they had an AMM and wanted to come see who it was. I guess AMM was stamped on my forehead after all. Can we say circus act? That is exactly how I felt at that moment. I heard the bullhorn say "Stay tuned to the ring master for more stunning performances by our new oddity, a rare case of AMM!"

Pain and exhaustion will certainly color a meeting. I had a bitter taste in my mouth after that; I don't know why. The fly under the microscope deal, maybe. Seems they were looking at all of my pieces yet not seeing me. Very uncomfortable, I realized my medical rollercoaster had left the station now and the biggest hill out there was a killer.

After 48 hours of sporadic sleep, I was able to sit up and move about a little easier. I ate something that was supposed to be eggs. Jack, Becky and Larry had gone home. On the third day Mom and Laura took me home to wait for my future.

I had an abdominal drain in place, could not walk upright, and was very tired. I spent most of my day on the couch but I moved around the house (having learned the lesson of inactivity so many years ago) trying to regain my mobility and strength. Laura nursed my wound and emptied my drain, keeping account of the type and amount of fluid that was present for Dr. Chapman's records. Laura stayed with me for a few days and kept me laughing through the pain.

One evening we were watching TV and an ad for the movie *The Nutty Professor* with Eddie Murphy came on the screen. The clip was the scene where his lips start to grow. Laura looked at me; tears were rolling down my face, fighting so hard to hold back those painful convulsions of laughter. Laura looked away from me and tried to stop but we could not stop! The more it hurt, the harder we laughed, truly laughing through the pain. Laura left the next day. I missed her. Nobody on this earth can make me laugh like Laura.

Two or three weeks later I returned to Vanderbilt to have the incision checked and the drain removed. Don and Mary drove me to Nashville this time as my appointment time was for 9:15 a.m. CST and I was much too tired and weak to do this trip alone. My recovery seemed to be a very slow one. Energy was a commodity I could not waste. Other people were required; I was blessed to have them available to help.

The area in my abdomen where the drain had been placed had started to become painful as the drain coming out of my abdomen was attaching itself to my body; every move stung. I was so looking forward to saying goodbye to the last remnant of my spleen removal.

The nurse called me back and put me into the same room that only a month or so before had been the site of my first major medical decision. The door popped open and Dr. Chapman came in.

"Okay, Janet, lie down on the table; we are going to get this drain out of your abdomen. I need you to take a deep breath and hold it until I tell you to slowly let it out."

With only a partial count he just yanked and out it came.

Well, Dr. Chapman, deep breath or no that removal hurt! However, the pain was fleeting and now that the drain was gone, I felt great. The incision was healing as expected.

In June, I tried to go back to work. I tried and failed on a regular basis. I was so tired. On July 7th, 2001, I gave up the ghost. Admitting I could not practice anymore was the most difficult realization I have ever had to accept. This was the first real declaration I was losing this battle with AMM. The scorecard would be lopsided for quite a while, I thought.

The clinic owner told me not to worry about work.

"The job will be waiting for you when you get through it all."

"It may be a while," I said with an, "are you sure" kind of look.

"I know, don't worry about your job." Doc walked away.

I wanted to believe that would be the case, but I did not really find much hope or comfort in the statement. Promises quickly made out of the emotion for any situation are the ones most often broken at the end of that journey. I could only hope Doc meant what was said that afternoon.

CHAPTER TWENTY-SEVEN

"This is Social Security, how may I help you?"

Before entering the hospital to have the spleen removed, my future inability to work had to be addressed. A veterinary education consumes many dollars, and those dollars come from several places: personal savings, loans and, if you are young enough, your parents. Since I was a "woman growed" upon embarking this endeavor, loans and personal savings footed the bill.

Working as a veterinarian brings a whole new reality in terms of financial future or possibility of the lack of one. Most of us are lucky in that our employers pay for some of our professional outlay. Some, is the operative word; we have fees, medical and liability insurances, organizational and state dues, continuing education costs, professional taxes and life in general to cover. We are not as well-paid as human doctors but our professional life is rewarded in other ways.

Graduation brings "good deals" to all students from our national membership organization the AVMA. One was a disability policy. In the middle of my first working year after school, it became apparent I could not pay for the policy (which, since I lived in Florida, was very expensive), pay back my school loans, my professional costs and have enough left over to put a roof over my head, clothes on my back, food in my mouth, and gas in my car. Something had to go and the choice was not an easy one. I dropped the policy; realized disability was tied to the health insurance policy that came as the other side of the deal, and lost both. I reapplied to BC/BS medical and they took me back and at a much lower rate than my so-called good deal. By the end of the story disability insurance was important but in this moment a non-starter. I would revisit it in the future.

Time passing allowed me to start saving some money and paying back my loans. By the time this disease became apparent about nine years later I still had some of my school loan left to repay and a nearly paid car loan. If no income was coming in, and with medical bills ensuing, what little savings I had would soon be consumed.

By splenectomy time, that was the case. The job I took after leaving Mark did not pay as well, so much of what had to be paid medically was starting to come out of savings. By April of 2001, the balance was dwindling. Help would be needed and I firmly believed it was not my family's job to take care of me. (Boy, did I underestimate them on that thought.) The illness journey meant not working, so no income. I had to apply for Social Security disability benefits. I had never been able to revisit the disability issue; the cost still was prohibitive for me to purchase a policy.

A more difficult request was hard to imagine for a woman who had worked hard to get farther and was now found the last horse in the race. Picking up the phone to tell the government I needed what I had paid in over the last 20-25 years, at first glance left me feeling that I had failed myself. Never mind that other people seem to turn their noses up when they find you are on disability. Seems they never really listen as to the why of the situation. Apparently, I was having the same attitude toward myself! This attitude was soon replaced with the reality of illness and disability.

The realization of sickness and a subsequent inability to work is not a moral failing. Fate has dealt you a hand, a bad circumstance, which is all it means. The stigma associated with the word disability needs to be gone. A person can only do what they can when they can. As working Americans we've already earned this insurance; we are just withdrawing the account. The only failure in this scenario was my ailing body. I am so very grateful the money was there to receive.

An appointment for a phone interview with the local SSA office was arranged. The day came, they called me at home, and we filled out the forms over the phone. The man on the other end indicated that with my medical status there should be no problem.

He told me, "This is why we have disability insurance. Dr. Smith, I know you will easily be approved."

Decisions usually required two to three months before a notification. All of my expenses were streamlined; only the necessities were budgeted. My family recognized my needs and my financial situation and eagerly helped where they could. My reserves were meager, a consequence of a midlife change in professions, but I felt I could pay what I had until I started to receive my disability benefits. This was around April of 2001.

CHAPTER TWENTY-EIGHT

"Poe's Raven gave up December rapping, transformed himself into Madan, and now was tap, tap, tapping on my iliac crest!"

The final ascent up the killer rollercoaster hill had begun. My choices were becoming fewer and much more focused. In July, I was to attend my CE with Ann and Traci. We were going to Boston this time.

I found it hard to believe that a year had passed since this journey had begun. Just barely under a year since that blue martini-washed talk with Traci occurred. So much had happened; so much of me had changed since then. My life was on a track I had no control over. I was a sick woman with only one goal: survive. I hoped my trip to Boston would not be my last trip ever. There were so many places I wanted to see on this old planet. But as it was I had to go see Vandy again. My world had collapsed to contain only my home, a car, the interstate to Nashville and back and the clinic at Vandy.

On June 20, 2001, I had to go to back to Vanderbilt to see Dr. Madan for a pre-transplant bone marrow tap, final blood work and a visit with radiology. My blood was getting more viscous since my splenectomy, my platelets were over 500,000, and my packed cell volume was hanging around 55 percent. I was taking hydroxyurea to slow down the cell production. Dr. Dobbs' office had been monitoring my counts and giving me phlebotomies since my spleen had been removed. I hoped the hydrea would not interfere with my transplant but I had no choice at this stage but to take the drug. My packed cells could not get too high and my platelets had to stay down to prevent clotting in my vessels.

Laura had to come back into town to have her final blood work completed. All data had to be obtained within 90 days of the transplant, put together in a package and sent to my insurance company for approval. My insurance was not paying for any of the donor testing costs. All came out of my pocket, for each of the siblings. At that moment, about 1500 dollars apiece times four. Oh, well, a way will show itself; I cannot go forward without the tests. All of the tests had to be run, the results acceptable and the information written up and sent to BC/BS in time.

I have a history of weak teeth. Dr. Mike Powers had been given the charge of keeping my mouth healthy enough for me to be transplanted.

Why do I keep hearing Paul Simon around all of these issues?

Bone marrow taps and spinal taps are traditionally given a high score on the patient fright scale. I had already had one in order to be diagnosed. Dr. Stein had done one after my splenectomy, I think. Now one more tap to endure before the big day. My anxiety about pain was a little more controlled that day. I chose to never again have sedation while having a bone marrow tap.

Laura had not seen me go through the procedure before that time. She sat in the chair next to the wall, was obviously worried for me and unsure of what to expect. So, she tried to make me laugh. What else is new?

Becky, was my nurse; her name was a comfort. The program began.

"Janet, lie on your stomach and if you need them grab the handles under the edge of the table."

My pants were lowered to below my pelvis. Becky prepped the site with Betadine scrub. After she draped me, she returned to the head of the bed. She began talking to me and rubbing my back, trying to ease any anxiety I may be having.

By then, Dr. Madan had arrived, and the lab technician had her prep plates ready to go.

"Hey, Janet, how are you?" Dr. J. walked over to the sink and washed his hands.

Madan is always cheerful, always smiling and ready to laugh.

"I'm OK, just want this over. Dr. J., I need you to look at my leg before you leave."

He said he would and got busy. He put his gloves on and began the procedure.

Dr. Jagasia has a wonderful touch with a tap. I have had two or three different doctors do them and Jagasia is the best. He realizes the pain and loads the site with lidocaine. Numbing the periosteum is so important. The covering of our bones is one of the most sensitive sites in the body, thus the pain of a broken bone. The periosteum is torn; that means pain. Taps enter the bone across the periosteum that means pain. The bone biopsy is worse than the marrow tap, at least for me.

The incision is made with a small stab over the iliac crest and the tap needle is pressed into the bone, into the marrow cavity. The stylet from the Jamshedi is removed and if blood rises, the marrow is accessed. If not, start again. The marrow is sucked out of the cavity with a syringe, like a big mosquito landing on your arm.

The pain runs up your back and down your legs and the degree of that pain is unpredictable so some taps are going to be worse than others. The main thing is they are tolerable with a little gritting of teeth, focused thought and controlled breathing, A good nurse to talk to you and take your mind off the procedure always helps. Of course, a little humor takes the edge off. I was so thin; my bones just popped out under my skin. I admonished Jagasia.

"Hey, Doc, take care and don't bend your needle on those bones!"

Madan just laughed and almost as in retribution for my bad joke put his weight behind the task of pushing that huge needle into my pelvis. Laura visibly contorted with imagined pain as she watched Madan laying his body weight onto the biopsy needle to take a piece of my bone. My body felt like it was being pressed into the very matrix of the metal table, like mercury, I became all oozing liquid and metallic.

The procedure was over soon enough. Laura began to see what my life had been since my initial diagnosis. Not too pleasant an existence. She told me after she hugged me that she had no idea how hard this has been for me to get through for the last year.

After the tap, my leg issue was addressed. The large vein that runs down the inside of my leg was inflamed from my groin down to my ankle. It was raised, red, blue, black, hot and painful. I could not walk without a limp; it stung with each muscle contraction. My blood was so thick and my platelet count so high I was getting inflammation of my vessels.

"Janet, let's get you some antibiotics. Should clear up, stay on your hydrea and recheck with Dr. Dobbs for a CBC in a couple of weeks." Madan wrote the script and said he would see me later.

"Thanks, Doc. See you later." Madan left the room and Laura went with nurse Becky to get more testing done. I had a date with radiology, in the basement of Vanderbilt.

The radiologist, a woman, was very nice and discussed the total body procedure that I would be given while being ablated for the transplant: Gamma rays, 1200 rads total dose, divided twice daily, for three days. Sounds easy enough just stand there twice a day for a few minutes. Piece of cake!

My body was measured by the technicians and I was told to let them know if, after my radiation, I had problems. I gathered my sister, left Vandy, went home and packed. I had a trip to take. I was going first class this time. It may be my last time.

Traci, Ann and I went to Boston and though I was painful and limping had a great time. We spent many of the early moments talking about my situation and how I was handling the stress. They were telling me how strong I was and how I had such a good attitude and how I was handling the uncertainty so well. Finally, I just asked them to stop. I appreciated their confidence in me but it was hard enough living with this thing daily and this was a time to try to not think about what my future may or may not hold. I wanted to forget about it on this trip and just be me, not sick me. They finally realized that and let it go.

As we left Boston, knowing there was a period of time or two I might be alone during treatment, I asked my friends if they might be able to come to Nashville for only a couple of days and help. I told them the apartment would be available and the trip would not cost them much cash. They could probably drive up together since Mobile was not that far away and save money on air fare as well.

Ann immediately said, "Yes, just let me know what you need. I would be more than happy to help."

Traci had a look of uh-oh on her face and without much feeling told me her position.

"I have already made plans and paid the money for a three-day event during that time frame; sorry. I will call and check on you."

I tried not to let my shock at her choice show on my face. I was a little stunned at her choice of a horse show several months away, especially after her response in Toronto. I had never asked anything much of my friends. I do not like to impose my needs on others. Guess that attitude just got reinforced.

Oh, well, live long enough and you will see everything, I guess. It struck me as how amazing it is that one simple conversation, one choice, can make one collate a past and thus alter a perception in a moment.

Reality lesson; we are present in life for what we value.

CHAPTER TWENTY-NINE

"What was that line? Oh yeah, some folks' lives"

Early in the transplant approval process, my insurance company, BC/BS of Tennessee, called to discuss the program's plan. I picked up the phone on the first ring.

"Hello?"

A very cheery male voiced asked.

"Is Ms. Janet Smith there, please?"

"Yes, this is she."

"Janet, this is Arthur Terry of BC/BS, and I have been designated as your transplant medical coordinator."

He seemed a pleasant man.

"Well, nice to make your acquaintance, Mr. Terry." I had never spoken with my insurance company rep.

"Janet, I need to discuss a situation around your transplant."

Arthur had that tone.

"Really, what situation is that?"

All I heard was "Some folks' lives'..."

"I need to explain to you that Vanderbilt is not on our transplant preferred provider list."

A quiet that passed all understanding developed on both ends of the connection. Vanderbilt was not on their list of preferred transplant centers. That refrain went through my head like that song I can't forget. Vanderbilt is not on our preferred providers list for transplants. How many ways could one patient hear that their insurance was not going to cover the transplant if they chose Vanderbilt?

How could the "Harvard of the South," one of the foremost research and medical facilities in the States, let alone Tennessee, not be on their list? I was stunned into near silence and after a moment of unbelieving I spoke.

"Arthur, you're kidding me, right?"

"No, Janet, I am not kidding."

I was sitting on my chair amazed, shaking my head, physically shaking, becoming nauseous and wondering what I was going to do now.

"Janet, there is some information about your choice I need to give you. BC/BS will only pay 60 percent of all incurred expenses if you choose to continue with Vanderbilt as your center."

I was looking at 250-500,000 dollars or more over the next three to four years, if I survived that long. I had already run through most of what I had been able to save. I could not work and would not ask my siblings to float this cost out of their pockets. They had families; I was not their responsibility. This debt would be insurmountable in my lifetime.

My next life choice had come quickly and on my blind side. I had to decide how I would deal with the degree of indebtedness a transplant would bring without full insurance coverage. I did not hesitate on the decision; my instincts told me what I had to do and I listened.

"Arthur, I do not care. I have already lost a wonderful doctor in Steve Wolff and a wonderful doctor in Tracy Dobbs, I have found a wonderful new doctor in Madan Jagasia and I am not going to give up Vanderbilt and the relationship I have developed with my transplant team. I have no intentions of running off to some other state to have this done. Won't happen."

I was still shaking, scared to death about the choice that had forced itself on my life. They had to understand I did not want to leave the state to have this done. Money, or lack of it, was one setback I just could not deal with over the long term. Would I let the lack of funds keep me from trying to survive? Could I leave my family with a huge debt if I did and died? Just how much could I expect? The questions came at me like machine gun fire. I had to get this settled today. Consequences be damned. Brain, shut up! Focus.

"OK Janet, what we can do is to try to develop a one-time contract with Vanderbilt to cover the cost at a pre-set price."

"Wonderful Arthur, let's do that then. Thanks."

Blessed again, BC/BS has come through for me when I needed them every time. I felt the tide had turned. Now it was the old adage of "Time" again. I had to wait to see if Vanderbilt and BC could get their ducks in a row. I had faith they would; they had to have done this before. The response about a single contract had been too forthcoming for it not to be routine. Right?

It was July 2001 and the approval process was aimed at a September time frame. At the end of August, the deal worked out and the date was set, September 15, 2001.

I would have a Hickman catheter placed into my chest on the 14th and enter the transplant ward on the 15th. Becky had begun making arrangements for the housing and care schedule I would need for the three months after the transplant long before a date was set. The social services at Vanderbilt helped her find locations and helped define my future needs. Blue Cross helped her define what they would pay for after the transplant as to food and apartment cost re-imbursement. Becky created a timetable for caretakers with the siblings and my cousin Mary so that I would never or would rarely be alone. (I ended up being by myself for about a week and a half overall, I think.)

The medical siblings would be with me right after the transplant and again as I first entered the apartment. Money was in place and I was prepared mentally and spiritually to take the journey toward ridding myself of AMM. My only job during this ordeal, survive, and if not that, prepare my soul to leave this earth behind.

I felt the need to tell my siblings and my mom what they meant to me and how they had influenced my life. I needed to let them know how much I loved them before I may not be able to tell them. Before the transplant, I wrote each a letter. Now, if I died, I could do so knowing that they would know how they had affected my life; what joy they were to me in this world. I read each to myself and felt even then I had woefully underrepresented their place in my life. The point was I tried.

CHAPTER THIRTY

"You have 14 days"

Shortly after I had applied to Social Security for my benefits, a letter arrived in the mail.

We are informing you that you are not considered disabled by our guidelines. If you feel this conclusion has been incorrectly reached you may appeal. The appeal papers are enclosed. You have 14 days from the date the letter was dated to fill out these forms and return them to our agency."

Fourteen days seemed time enough. I looked at the date on the letter and the date of the postmark. I learned very quickly that SS always write letters on Monday, posts them in batch on Friday and by the time you receive the letter, you usually have less than a week to fill the papers out and get them returned. What a joke.

I had a terminal disease, and I had sludge for blood. Scheduled to undergo an allogenic transplant in a couple of months, I would not be able to be around people without risk for at least four months. I would be lucky to get back to part-time work in a year. But, the government said I was not disabled and could work. Boy, that piece of knowledge was so comforting; to know they had so much faith in me. How could I have doubted myself so?

I filed the request for review. This was the middle of August 2001. What a birthday present!

CHAPTER THIRTY-ONE

"Now who's rap, rap, rapping at my door? Murphy?"

Sleep was not something I could depend on and I was usually up by 6 a.m. This day was no different. The morning of September 11, 2001 found me sitting at my computer checking my messages. NBC's *Today Show* was quietly playing in the background. Around eight o'clock or a little after, I began hearing screams and sounds of disbelief coming from the TV behind me. I looked around to see the second plane hit a fiery World Trade Center.

"Mother! My God! Look at this!"

Mom hurried into the room and was stunned at the sight on the tube.

"What has happened here?"

"Planes are crashing into the trade towers. I can't believe this!"

In that moment I traveled two different experience trails. One was the day the Challenger exploded, the next took me back to the night Dad and I watched CNN as we invaded Iraq the first time. Watching bombs fall on Baghdad was unexpected that night and like that night I was speechless; the horror of what had just occurred sent strong feelings of loss and revulsion through my body and mind.

This time, it was my country. The trade towers were ablaze and falling. People were dying. America attacked in a way that definitely got our attention. How could anyone do such a deed? This time Paul Simon was speaking for us all.

CHAPTER THIRTY-TWO

"What did Laura say? She was the property of the United States government?"

As the day wore on, my realization that this attack was no little problem for the United States or for my life hit home and hit hard. Plane travel was at a standstill. Our nation was at the highest state of alert. My donor was in the military. What was going to happen this time? My brother Larry was in surgery and made the statement that events like these affect us all; my sister's transplant is this week.

I called Laura and was lucky to get through before she was isolated to the base.

"Laura?"

"Sis, I can't talk now. I have to get my bag in the car and get to the base. We have to get ready for casualties."

"Nell, the transplant is this week, are they going to let you go? What can we do? When will you know? Are we going to have to use Jack as the donor?"

"I don't know yet, Sis; I will talk to my commander as soon as I can. The base is at highest alert; there are tanks and machine guns everywhere. I don't know what will happen. I'll call when I can, bye."

Laura hung up. I had no idea when or if I would or could speak to her again. The transplant was to occur in four days. Laura was out of touch and my life was to be put in that oh so familiar hold pattern of time once again.

I was in a total fear mode. I called Jack in Atlanta.

"Jack Smith."

"Jack? You may have to be my donor if Laura cannot get out of Virginia."

Jack recognized the fear of uncertainty in my voice. Jack, like Becky, does not do medical well. His response was a tentative "Okay, what do I need to do? I'm here, let me know."

"I'll call as soon as I know. Bye, Jack."

I don't know what I was thinking. Laura was my best donor. Like me, she had never been pregnant, was younger than me, and she was a 6/6 HLA match. The chance for GVH would be lower with Laura.

Reality check, Janet. Jack had not been tested within the allotted time frame for the transplant. He could not step in at the last moment and be my donor. Fate must shine through or who knew when or if I would be transplanted.

After I had hung up from speaking to Jack, all I could think of, in spite of the horror our nation had just suffered, was would she get here? Would they let her come? What is it with this disease journey and its persistent ability to create havoc on plans and demand more and more time and space to interfere?

I had myself mentally prepared, schedules were in place. I called Dr. Madan; his nurse answered. I told her about the situation with Laura. She said she would talk to Dr. J. The nurse hung up and called me back an eternity later.

"Janet, maybe you should wait."

Did she not realize what she had just asked of me? Was she just oblivious or what? These words were Madan's but I could not believe they were real.

"No! I'm ready to do this thing, now! Psychologically, spiritually and financially ready to do this thing. People and schedules are in place. I don't want to wait any longer. How can I?"

I was determined to do this during this window of opportunity. If I had to wait, I was not sure how strong I still would have been medically, psychologically or spiritually when the actual time did come to begin the procedure. The first preparation was difficult enough: the medical toll of removing my spleen was becoming a player and I was not so sure I had the mental strength to attain this level of sureness and peace again. What if Laura was deployed in the future? How much toll the disease would take by the next possible date pervaded my thoughts. The possibility of my disease process going out of control and converting to an acute leukemia (a terminal step) worried me more than my self preparation. I could control me; I could not control my bone marrow.

My bone marrow was making those fibrocytes like crazy and they were pushing my immature little cells out of the nest way too soon. I didn't have a spleen anymore to deal with that overflow. This disease was out of control. I was at peace spiritually for the moment, but life sure can rile things up at times.

"I'll have Dr. Jagasia call." She hung up.

In a few moments, I heard Madan's voice, I knew he was smiling, I could hear it as he said my name.

"Janet I hear you are ready to do this."

"Yes, I and those around me are ready; I don't want to wait." I then heard the smile disappear from Madan's voice.

"Janet, unless Laura is attached to your side when you come in the hospital door I cannot ablate you. We cannot do this on a chance she will be here. Maybe we should put it off. You have some time."

There's that damn word again. I knew the treatment could not start without her; once started you cannot stop. However, I had faith it would work out and I did not want him to change plans yet. So, I begged him, an activity that would soon become an integral part of my nature.

"Please, give me time to see if Laura can get here; if anything her situation is only going to get worse! She's military! This may be the only time for a long time."

"I hadn't thought about that possibility. Keep me informed; I won't change any of the plans." This was late in the day of September 11.

I hung up the phone from speaking with Madan and called Becky. I was scared to death. What if Laura cannot get here, what am I going to do? This was the first time I had actually felt a degree of panic around my disease control plan. Larry was right. It seems the events of that morning were going to affect many more lives in this nation, one way or another. Becky started calling airlines trying to determine if Laura could be flown down. Delta said drive.

Laura called the next morning, September 12.

"Sis, my superiors are working on getting me out."

"What do you think? Will they OK this a second time?"

"I don't know, Sis, I will let you know." She hung up. Limbo was still the game.

I was very nervous, praying all the time. I was so prepared to do this now. I could not imagine having to wait. When one has prepared for the worst and hopes for the best and then that resolve is put into jeopardy, fear runs rampant. I was afraid I would never be as ready to do this as I was at this moment. Deep down though I was recognizing a peace and calm that silently, at first imperceptibly, was taking over my body. In that moment I knew, I knew that an answer would be in my favor. I started to relax and early on September 13, Laura called.

"I am packing the car. Col. Sewall said since it was life or death and they had already approved the time, they would let me go."

"Thank you, God, be careful, Sis. We will see you this afternoon." I hung up.

Blessed again! The trip from Bowie to Rockwood was about 13 hours. She drove into the driveway late that afternoon. Becky was already home when Laura came through the door. Hugs were many and long.

My appointment for the Hickman catheter placement was not until later in the day of the 14th. That catheter would be the method all my chemotherapy agents would be given. That morning we packed the cars with all of my stuff and having called Dr. Madan to confirm, left Rockwood.

I was reliving the day I left home to start college. The emotion was overwhelming; tears cascading down my cheeks from behind my sunglasses. College meant I was able to come home anytime I wanted. This journey gave no guarantees. I was leaving behind all I held dear. The exception being my family; they would be with me.

I looked back over my shoulder as we drove away. Would I ever see my home again? Laura and I drove up in her car; we talked some, laughed a lot and tried to stay positive about the next few weeks. Mother and Becky followed. I did not want Mom to watch me go through this procedure. I could not keep her away.

The placement of the Hickman was done under heavy sedation. I remember waking up from time to time but do not remember anything other than moving bodies and a green room.

When the catheter was in place, I went to recovery where Mom and Laura were waiting. Becky was out checking on last-minute details on the apartment and tying up other loose ends. We went back to the hotel room, met up with Becky, ate dinner and waited for the next day.

CHAPTER THIRTY-THREE

"We are healed of a suffering only by experiencing it to the full."

Marcel Proust

The elevator dumped us out onto the hallway connecting the transplant and neurology wards. The neuro ward waiting room was right in front of us.

Frightened, pacing, scared, mourning people were waiting, wrapped in warm hospital blankets, wrapped in each other's arms, contorted into shapes that allowed them to sleep in the lounger chairs; waiting in warm, dimmed light and deathly quiet except for the ubiquitous TV, the occasional pop, pop, pop, of, weirdly enough, popcorn cooking in the microwave, the transient odor of old pizza and the inevitable screams of loss. My heart sank. I looked at my sisters and my mom. I know I had fear in my eyes. They were looking at me, obviously afraid for me with what was just around the bend, my treatment, my walk to death and back.

"Let's go." I put the scene in the past.

That much fear, sorrow and worry was not what I needed right now as it was vital to stay positive. We turned to the left and around the bend. Laura pushed the vacuum door button that was on the wall, opened the air lock doors, and we arrived on the transplant ward, 11 North. The atmosphere on this ward was as warm and bright and hopeful as the neuro ward had not been in just the brief moment before. The floor receptionist smiled as if she had known me all my life and spoke with a cheery tone as we strolled in with all my paraphernalia.

"Hello, Ms. Smith. You are to go to room 25. Your nurse will be there in a moment."

"OK, thank you; which way?"

"Straight down the hall to your right, last door on the left."

"Thanks."

We headed down the hall toward my new and possibly last home. I stopped that train of thought, realizing one more time since entering the hospital that I could not think in those terms. I must stay focused and positive and survive. So it was resolved that 11025 would be my home for a simple 30-day stint.

There was a can of spray disinfectant on the wall outside the room. We opened the door and walked into this little niche numbered 11025 to find empty walls painted off-white and a window looking out toward the hospital garage and one near the door looking onto the ward, a bath with a shower, a sink in the room, a closet and a TV/VCR. Of course we found the standard hospital bed with railings and a remote control for the nurse, the bed, and the TV.

The moment caved in again. I saw the walls move toward me, the air was heavy with a pungent odor. Why didn't my sisters and Mom notice it? They were busily setting my belongings on the floor, laughing and taking measure of where to put everything I had dragged along from home.

Again, that black hole named fear was lurking on the fringes and survival demanded refocusing on the moment. I couldn't allow anything getting ahead of the actions of getting settled in my room and starting my treatment. That was all I had to do today. They were not difficult or fearful tasks. So, I reacted to my family's lead.

"I'm glad we brought my room stuff from home. I don't want to spend the next 30 days in an old sterile hospital room. I need my things and pictures of my family around me."

We had lugged my books, music, photos, clothes, quilt and pillow and transplanted anything that meant anything to me from home into Vanderbilt Hospital. The only thing I could not bring, my dogs.

Several days before leaving for Vanderbilt, I took my precious cocker spaniels, Topper and Heather, to stay with Susan and David Porterfield, in Knoxville. I cried like a baby as I handed Susan their leashes. I was so afraid that I would never again see Susan or my dogs.

"Thanks for taking care of them for me Susie; if I die, please make sure they are taken care of, OK?"

Susan grabbed me and held on, tears rolling down our cheeks.

"They will be fine and so will you; I can't lose one of my best friends. You'll be back, don't worry and I will write and call."

"I love you too, and I'll do what I have to do to get back here. Mom will pick them up when she comes back home after phase one."

"Not a problem; they can stay as long as they need to, we love them as our own."

"I'll never be able to repay your kindness, Susan."

"You can, just get through this."

Walking out that door left me crushed, tears rolling down my cheeks. The pain was breathtaking. I had just left a huge part of myself in that grooming shop. Regaining that part of me was now a major survival goal.

Carol Sanders was my charge nurse. She watched as we hauled all that stuff into 25, one of the smaller rooms on the ward. She took the measure of the situation and decided my room was too small. Carol stuck her head in the door.

"Janet, would you like a bigger room if one opens up?"

"Absolutely, if that can be done, that's great!"

I wondered what "opened up" meant. Would somebody die or go home?

I didn't want to know the answer. I entered the ward on a day with two other patients; would the 33 percent chance rule hold? Would I be the one to survive? I prayed for all of us to break the rules, and was determined to go through this with a smile and the quiet determination to survive.

We began to put my things in closets but thankfully never finished. About an hour later, Carol comes in the room smiling about her news.

"Let's go!"

Laura, Becky and Carol carted all of my room stuff down the hall to room 11023, home for the next 30 days. We unloaded again.

"Sis, where do you want the book stand?" Laura had her hands full.

"Where I can see it from my bed." Laura, put it underneath the TV stand. "That's good."

"Jan, where do you want these clothes?" Becky had two bags in her hands.

"In the closet, I'll hang them up later."

Mom sat down next to the window. She let her girls sort this out.

"View isn't bad, you can see downtown Nashville."

Mom had staked her claim to the ever-present hospital room lounger chair. Opening her bag, taking out her pencil and her crossword puzzle she started filling in the words. Mom was happy. Becky, Laura and I finished getting me settled. About and hour later the door popped open.

"OK Ms. Janet, let's get you started."

Carol and Teresa had gifts of drugs, urinary catheters, and fluids. IV poles and pumps were to be bedside companions for the duration. The grim reaper, or maybe the Countess Dracula of Bone Marrow; had just arrived in the form of a very nice, blond-headed nurse; it didn't matter the name. Those drugs she was purveying were my approach to death.

"Carol, what is all that?"

"Cytoxan, saline, and a foley; we have to monitor your urine for blood. Cytoxan can cause your bladder to bleed. We also need to make sure you are producing enough urine."

"Lovely, I'm looking forward to that!"

Mom and the sisters left to get some lunch and to get into the apartment. Draculetta began invading my body.

"Janet, the ablation starts today. Cytoxan is going to make you sick. Let me know when you feel nauseous and the doctors have something ordered I can give you. Radiation will start in a day or so."

Carol kept talking to me. As she kept busy with the lines, meters and drugs I put on my life jacket, stepped into my boat and started my journey down the river Styx. The current was gentle, lulling me into a sense of trust and calm. The magic involved with the exposure of the process and the busy work around it tried to hide the fact that my death cruise had begun.

All of the preparatory months, prior to this one moment, had been couched in the luxury of "not yet." "Not yet" was here. I looked at my family photos, blinked away my tears, prayed for strength, grace and peace for all involved and began my internal war with the unknown rapids ahead that could capsize my desire for survival. Never mind that the boat carrying this whole show could fail outright; it was all such a risk no matter how many times Vandy had done this treatment. The river flowed on.

The evening jump started with a buzz to the nurse's station just across the hall. Carol wasted no time.

"Yes, Janet, what do you need?"

"I'm nauseous." Carol nodded her head and started to leave.

My mouth was full of warm, voluminous, thick, slimy mucous. It was almost like snails had filled my mouth with their slimy trails. Disgusting! I hate to vomit. My stomach began to contract and here it came propelling itself up my esophagus, squeezing itself through my nose and spewing out of my mouth all hot, burning and full of my last lunch. Chemo vomit spread slowly all over the floor, under my bed and onto my shoes, splashing my sheets and pajamas with little chemo polka dots; just volumes of vomit. Round one: A TKO by Cytoxan and several more rounds were its to win as well. I did not have any training to beat this foe. This drug was out to kill me off and only my doctors could get its attention long enough to distract it from the job.

"Let me clean that up, Janet, and we'll get you something. How about phenagren? Let's see how it works first." Carol's suggestion meant little.

"Fine, whatever. I don't care; just make it go away." Curling into a ball, I tried to go to sleep. No luck there either. Carol came back into the room.

"Janet, do you want a popsicle or some Jello?"

Carol knew the routine. She had been giving support, confidence and stability to people on the floor for many years. I was grateful to have her around.

"I love Jello; sure, I'll try it."

After a few more rounds of vomiting warm liquid Jello up my esophagus through my nasal passages and over my taste buds, I developed a definite distaste for any foodstuff that giggles, is brightly colored and melts into a burning acidic rerun. Eventually, the phenagren did not do much to stop the vomiting and the best drug for me was Zofran.

Dr. Madan was not on my rotation, I knew that, but was a little disappointed. Doctors Greer and Morgan were on rotation during my stay on the ward. I was to depend on doctors I did not know, and who did not know me. Maybe that was the plan, no preconceived ideas or pre-existing relationships. Maybe this protects the doctors too. That floor has its share of bad days for everyone.

The morning of the second day, my exam indicated an increase in lung sounds. Did I have pneumonia already? That was Becky and Laura's cue to become activity coordinators.

One of Becky's friends had had an auto transplant. Mary, like David, had had lymphoma. She told Becky many things to look for with me, and an exercise routine was very important. I had to establish a daily routine, no matter how sick I felt. Becky was not going to let me forget Mary Nagashige's advice.

They really thought they would have to make me get up and moving. Not so. Having had pneumonia while in vet school, one hint of that disease was incentive enough to get up and out the door. After I started walking every morning, I noticed that all of the women patients on the ward exercised every day, sometimes twice a day. Every morning our blinds were opened and the sun shone into our rooms, warm rays of hope.

The men, on the other hand, seemed to close the blinds, crawl into their beds, pull their covers up to their necks, sink into the TV and rarely make an appearance. I wondered how they stood the waiting that way, ostriches with their heads in the sand.

The second day started early. I was realizing sleep was not a priority on this floor; schedules were the motivation. Blood was pulled on schedule every morning at 3 a.m. Nurses' aides take vital signs every four hours. Treatments come early in the morning and by mid-afternoon.

Radiation therapy for transplant is total body. Some cancers get local treatment. Transplants need total marrow destruction. The summer visit to Vandy gave radiation techs the opportunity to take my body measurements for the cage. Treatments began about 9:30 on the morning of the 16th with a knock on my door.

"Come in."

The door opened. "Ms. Smith?"

"Yes, come in."

A large, smiling, orderly in blue scrubs, driving a wheelchair was outside my door.

"No, I'll wait here. I'm to take you down for your radiation treatment, Ms. Smith."

"Oh, OK, just let me get my mask and my shoes and jacket." I had noticed I was starting to really feel the cold.

"I'll go with you, Sis."

Becky was afraid for me. I wanted them to know I had surrendered to this and was at peace with the ordeal I would suffer, whatever the outcome.

"OK, I'll enjoy the company while I wait my time in the queue."

We gathered my lines and bags of fluids, disconnected them from my chest catheter, and headed to the elevator. I couldn't leave the urine bag behind though; it was placed in my lap.

"Sis, I'll see you there." Becky turned toward the elevator by the neuro ward. We turned toward the dog leg in the hall, bearing right.

"Why aren't you going this way?"

"I can't, see you there."

My driver spoke.

"Ms. Smith, we'll go the back way, underneath the hospital so you won't be exposed to other people."

"Oh, I see."

The basement pathway was a hallway of painted cinderblocks and downward sloping concrete flooring. Dark, cold and foreboding, he wheeled me along the tunneled path and then the light from radiology became apparent about 500 feet ahead. Becky's outline was black, fully in front of the light filling the hallway.

My transport left me in the queue with a lot of other people, all just waiting. We all looked resigned to our fate, young and old. I saw the person in the room next to mine on a stretcher bed lined in the queue behind me. Rick had aplastic anemia. We nodded to each other; Becky introduced us. She and Laura had met Rick's wife and had met Rick.

The technician rolled me through a thick door. On my right, a huge piece of off-white equipment that bore an uncanny resemblance to a Krispy Kreme doughnut was in the middle of the room, a black frame stand on the wall opposite. The room was cinder block painted that odd hospital green. The room felt very cool. If I could have given it a human nature I would have said it was totally uncaring and narcissistic or was that just my fear trying to step into this play again?

The black metal stand had a bicycle seat in the middle and handles on either side. Placed in the cage, they told me to stand still and to not sit down unless I had to. The technicians moved the bars of the cage to my measurements and left the room. I heard a whir. I was to stand facing the front until they told me to turn.

I zoned out. My mind was not invited to these affairs. I can do mindless for six minutes, just focus on the task; get through it. Becky smiled as I left the room and met me back upstairs. I waited for the next treatment of the day, probably around 3 p.m. My first radiation treatment had made my temperature to rise. I did not feel very well; increasingly more tired and nauseous. Each bag of Cytoxan, each second in radiation, was removing my life, I felt each ounce lost.

The immediate reality was that the fluid lines and urinary catheter were already becoming nuisances. With every motion I had to clear lines or move the bag of urine. Going to the rest room was a major endeavor. The nurses set up my lines so to give me a lot of running room. It was still a cumbersome situation. Walking every morning around the halls of the unit, carrying a bag full of urine and pushing a pole full of fluid bags, pumps and lines was a real circus. You got past appearances real quick and became quite nimble, despite the bulk you had to carry along with you. Patience around all things new became a morning mantra for me now.

The afternoon of the first day of treatment, Laura and Becky were going to go to the gym at Vanderbilt and exercise. Mom was back at the apartment resting, watching her soaps. The family learned early that they had to take care of themselves to take care of me. For some reason though, Laura felt she should stay with me after that treatment. I knew it would not be comfortable for her in the reclining chair because her hips were painful from the Neupogen working on her bone marrow.

Beginning my first day of treatment, and for the next five days, Mother would give Laura daily injections of Neupogen. This drug causes the bone marrow to turn on and start making stem cells. When my marrow was dead, day five, the Red Cross would harvest the cells from Laura.

Laura had made herself as comfortable as she could in the chair. The TV had been turned off and my room was dark for once, the blinds closed. It was not yet shift change.

I got up, fluid lines tangled under my feet, and I fought my way into the bathroom. I regained control of the lines and clumsily wandered back, hung my urine bag on the side of the bed, crawled onto the mattress and I covered up; very cold. As I lie there, my chest began to feel full, and fluttery. I became lightheaded and nauseous.

"Nell?"

"Huh?" My cry had startled her. She had already succumbed to sleep, typical Laura. She can sleep standing up.

"My heart is weird; it feels like a bag of worms in there."

Laura, going instantly into her ER nurse mode, jumped up, forgetting her own pain and took my pulse, well over 180.

Seconds later the door yanked open.

"Carol, we need an EKG; Janet's rhythm or rate is off!"

Before I could sneeze there was a monitor going. Laura hooked this up, and a cardiologist consulted. It seems that the atria of my heart were a little irritable. High doses of chemotherapeutics can cause this problem. Cardizem was placed into my IV fluids. All quieted down and I went to sleep. Bullet number two dodged.

The next morning brought the man with the wheelchair bright and early. I was sick, very tired already and had no control over anything anymore; didn't care, really. I put on my mask and my sweatshirt, placed my head in my hands, told Becky and Laura I would see them later and took the ride down the elevator through the bowels of VUMC to the radiation treatment area. I had no idea that as I left my room and the door closed, Becky collapsed into tears and into Laura's arms; both found full of fear and concern for me. As they cried in my room, I entered the room of radiation.

"Good morning, Dr. Janet. Go ahead and step into the cage."

The techs came over to help me climb the step, realizing I was too weak to do it alone. My standing up left me quite seasick.

I'm gonna vomit!" I fell back into the wheelchair.

The technicians scattered away and out of range of the splatter. Chemotherapy vomit is full of toxins to normal people. Cleanup is a HAZMAT activity. The techs gave me an emesis bowl. I then stood up and headed back into the cage. Whirr.

"Three minutes, turn, please." My legs were gone. I had to lean on the seat. Whirr.

"Three minutes, and you are done."

Back to the chair, the orderly found me in the hallway. Vacant of thought, my body was completely exhausted. The last treatment had really taken me down the rabbit hole. I was ignorant of the path back through the bowels of Vandy, back up the elevator and into my bed.

That afternoon the whole episode repeated, vomit and all. This time I sat through the treatment. Thank God, it was over. I was so weak, and I just wanted to crawl in bed and sleep.

The third day of radiation therapy is still not registering in my mind as an occurrence. All I know is I got through it and survived the treatments one more time. I did not have to do it anymore. A few days after the radiation treatments Becky asked me, "Jan? Did you know the nurses call radiation the oven?"

"No, but I can see why, I have the best tan I have had in years."

We just hugged and laughed, easy to do when total body radiation therapy is behind you.

CHAPTER THIRTY-FOUR

"Finish each day and be done with it. You have done what you could. Some blunders and absurdities no doubt crept in; forget them as soon as you can. Tomorrow is a new day, begin it well and serenely and with too high a spirit to be cumbered with your old response."

R.W. Emerson.

Sunday afternoon in September in Middle Tennessee offers trees still green, air still warm and summer sweet, and people out in the last of the summer sun taking their typically Southern Sunday drives. Mom and Laura were with me that afternoon when a knock on the door broke the chatter.

"Come in."

"Hey! You aren't bald. I expected you to look near death!"

Dr. Eugene Kline and his wife had brought their sunshine to me.

I was so immunosupressed any germ could have killed me. Visitors were not high on my list of needs. Nonetheless, joy flooded my happiness circuits when Dr. Kline and his wife Ruth Ann walked in that Sunday afternoon.

"EK" is one of my lifetime touchstones. He has kept me in line since my graduate school days. He is tall, balding, a little round, jovial, unbelievably intelligent, spiritual and highly motivating. I love the blessing of Eugene Kline in my life.

"No, I am not bald yet, I've not been here a week." I knew he was thinking Janet, always the procrastinator.

"Well, you look good; not too sick?"

"I have my moments; maybe you won't see one while you are here!"

He and his wife laughingly agreed they could do well without an exhibition.

"It was such a beautiful day we thought we would take a drive after church and we decided we would come see you. I sure was hoping to see you bald!"

"Well, I'll send you a picture then."

"That will do."

"Dr. Kline, you remember my mom, Rosalie, don't you? My sister Laura took chemistry at Tech. I don't know if you knew her then or not."

"Yes, I do remember Mom. How are you, Mrs. Smith?"

Looking at Laura, "You did?"

"Yes, I had Dr. Swindell while I was getting my B.S. in nursing. I got through chemistry because Janet helped me nearly every night. Dr. Swindell said the difference between me and Janet was that Janet actually understood her chemistry."

We all laughed, with EK agreeing. "Yes, Janet did understand."

"Well, won't keep you; we just wanted to check in. We are going to get a bite to eat and head back to Cookeville. Keep me up to date."

"Becky will email you. Bye."

EK left a smile on my soul. Laura and Mom left to go to the apartment and eat.

Now that I was alone, the reality of the ward came crashing back into view. Solitude seemed to bring that reality nearer, more palpable than at any other time.

I was thankful I had my family around and the noise from the nursing station across the hall to keep the solitude at bay. Each voice I heard reminded me I was still a part of this old world, even though locked in the mostly sterile, highly-filtered, vacuum world of 11 North.

I could do nothing but move through this time moment to moment. Too much time to think about my therapy was not always a productive tool, but it seems it was one of the only tools I had. I could not read, had difficulty focusing, did not want food; I had walked the floors until a groove was forming, and I found just the occasional warm body to speak to me was comfort and distraction enough to get through each day.

When one is on a transplant ward, time to think helps one realize each new morning brings a day that divides itself into medical activity and the body's response to that activity. Nothing more or less of the physical world is brought with each new sun. The peripherals of the day remain the same: doctors, nurses, the occasional visitor, baths, food or lack of, phone calls, TV, prayers, schedules and lots of medicine.

The sometimes forgotten and often unrealized gift in those structured, passing days is the knowing that each day that passes brings a milestone. There are no "insignificant" days during a transplant, no matter how interminable or mundane they appear to the patient.

The spiritual aspect of life becomes the guide through these days, if one is open to the need of something other than the self. Meditation was for me an important part of those days. Staying focused on my job was my only hope and the only active participation I had during the treatment process.

Each day I awoke before dawn, opened the blinds and sat at the window, watching the sun come up over the Nashville skyline. Every morning was prayer-filled. Every morning found me thanking God for the success of yesterday and for the grace He would give me, my family and my team on that new day of rising. I would pray for strength to accept whatever outcome I would find at the end of the journey. Every day's end, I would watch the eastern horizon fade to deep blue as the sun faded out of the sky on its western traveling arc, finally dropping from the sky behind the hospital. Once again; I gave thanks.

CHAPTER THIRTY-FIVE

"Day zero and counting."

Five days into the journey and my bone marrow was dead. My white count had hit bottom, time for the transplant: DAY ZERO.

That morning, Laura and Becky had gone to the Red Cross blood unit, located across the street from the hospital. Laura had been prepped with a daily injection of Neupogen, a bone marrow stimulant. Time had come to reap the fruits of those shots.

Laura sat down in the lounger chair and the nurses put two fluid lines in her arms. The process would take three to four hours. Each drop of Laura's blood flowed from one arm, was filtered and the stem cells harvested. Her filtered blood went back into her other arm. She said there was no pain involved and she taught the nurses that, yes, you can go to the bathroom during this procedure!

Her cells were sent to the lab at Vanderbilt identified and counted. A normal harvest will yield around three to four million cells. Less than that count and the transplant may not succeed.

The day was gorgeous, sunny, glowing, and I was sitting on my bed talking to Mother, waiting for the cells, when Laura and Becky marched into the room. As the girls arrived; Carol came in with my new life in her hands. I believe Dr. Morgan was with her.

"You ready? Here they are, and quite a large number of them, I might add."

Carol laughed. Laura, in true style, made double the minimum amount of cells. Go, Nell!

"Janet, this will be really anticlimactic."

Carol checked the label on the bag of cells against my name bracelet and double checked my blood type, turned and hung the bag of pinkish-white liquid on the pole beside my bed as she had all the other bags of fluids and drugs.

Life started seeping into my blood stream as Carol opened the roll valve on the line. Soon all those little stem cells would respond to the chemotactic signals and factors that our body uses to tell cells to what part of the body they should go. In about 13 days they should find my marrow space and start to set up house.

For each up moment, there is, according to the laws of nature, a down side. The down side to this day was that I knew Laura's stem cells would find a new home only if the myelofibrosis had not scarred my marrow cavity too badly and only if Laura's cells decided they were a part of me after all. Those events were the unknowns in the equation. Again, only time would deliver the answer.

The empty bag of stem cells meant my 100 days were here, the next leg of my journey. These next three months would bring one of three outcomes: cure, a new disease process secondary to the treatment, or no implantation and death.

The first mile marker: implant.

Heavy, stomach-churning, bile-tinged fear was oozing around my room that morning, looking for any weak seal to enter and take hold of our hope. I had reached the point of no return. The category five rapids on the river Styx, that I so feared, were looming large in my foreground. I could only lie there, let the river current happen, and hope my life force had the strength to fight the pull and turn to another less dangerous rivulet. Failing that, I prayed I had garnered the experience and the grit from a lifetime of trials to make it through the roughest shoot.

Laura is not much of a crier, unlike Becky and me. Looking over at Laura from my bed and seeing her face contorting, and watching her tears streaming from those steel-blue eyes and down her reddening face, really hit me hard. In that moment we all recognized how all of the unspoken wishes, all of the fears of failure and all of Laura's personal stresses from knowing she was the only one who could possibly save my life hit home in a nanosecond. Laura managed her words of hope through her welling emotions generated from a year's worth of preparation and stress.

"I love you Sis; I pray my cells work."

We all had tears filling our eyes by now. Those warm, blessed tears of hope began running down on our cheeks and washing the fear of failure out of the room.

Dr. Morgan left the room post-haste; he seemed uncomfortable with the emotional display. He could have just left to give us our moment; one never knows with men.

"I love you too, Nell, and they will work."

Taking each other's hand, we then hugged. Becky hugged Mom and Carol wiped her own tears off her cheek. We remembered my first day here, holding hands and making the pledge to one another that we would fight this disease together and beat it. Our goal had not changed.

Tears did not last long; seems they never do in our family. Fear tears were soon laughing tears as Laura piped up with a prediction of my future.

"Next time I see you, you will be a "Chia Head!" And you will be craving chocolate pie and green beans!"

"I don't think so, Sis! Never, never, never. Ick!"

"Oh, I'll be sending thought waves to you from Maryland, telling my cells they need it. They'll hold you hostage until you eat chocolate pie or green beans."

"Well, I guess I'll die then. Visions of you poking green beans down my throat would be enough to push me over the edge."

Hope amplified filled the room. Mom, Laura and Becky left the next day and Larry came on line before the week was out.

CHAPTER THIRTY-SIX

"Pray and let God worry"

Martin Luther

The vestiges of AMM were pressing in around me, deciding whether it was letting me live or die. My soul was watching the story unfold, seemingly unconcerned. Hovering around me as a hummingbird in a safe place, my soul was free from fear, free from concern, and at total peace.

My body though was past exhaustion. All it wanted and needed was sleep and quiet. That was the impossible dream. The door opened, it was Carol again.

"Hey, you look great. I just know you are going to make it. We have new drugs today."

"Glad you have such faith in my tired old body's ability. What drugs?"

"Cyclosporine, methotrexate."

"What are they for?"

"They help your body accept the graft, high doses of immunosuppressants."

"What side effects this time?"

"Well, the methotrexate can cause oral ulcers, mucositis can worsen. The cyclosporine can cause an increase in blood pressure, loss of magnesium and kidney problems. Other things too; let's not worry about that now. You need to start using those mouth washes on a daily basis."

Dr. Madan had mentioned all of these factors to me at that meeting before my splenectomy. I suppose my vacuum tube environment did not allow me to hear too well, a need to recognize-only basis ruled the infiltration of my brain the day we discussed transplant side effects.

The pendulum of time was swinging again and the family had no idea if, when or where it would stop. Would I have life or death, health or some form of continued illness? Now the medical goals had changed from marrow destruction to marrow recovery. My medicine cabinet was already full. Daily protocol consisted of chemotherapeutic drugs, antibiotics, anti-virals, anti-fungals, anti-nausea, anti-acid, and anti-depressants. Most of these were IV drugs since I could not swallow very well. When mucositis starts, mouth washes help to stop oral ulcers from getting worse by keeping oral disease causing agents down in number.

Morphine will control the pain. Once mucositis starts, it continues to worsen until your epithelial cells lining your mouth and gut regenerate, usually 10-14 days. Two weeks of pain begins, along with not wanting anything in your mouth except cold water, popsicles and milk shakes. I enjoyed instant breakfast, chocolate. I do not know how I handled such strong, acidic flavors.

IV cyclosporine causes an elevation in blood pressure and can alter kidney function. I started on Norvasc to keep my blood pressure normal and Lasix to keep my urine flowing. Magnesium was added to my fluid therapy as the cyclosporine also causes you to lose it into your urine.

Over time, cyclosporine caused my eyes to focus poorly and my hands to shake. On days plus-three, six and eleven, I was given Methotrexate. This drug always made me feel worse. My throat would ulcerate more, I would have no desire to eat because of the pain of swallowing, and nausea worsened. I would even have diarrhea sometimes.

I was resisting morphine until one day Dr. Greer, in his typical forthright manner, told me a secret.

"Janet, we don't give medals around here for people in pain."

Well, that told me morphine was coming. Morphine shut down my intestinal tract. That meant laxatives were added to all the other indignities. Dr. Greer liked to remind me he had a goodly supply of soap if I needed it. I said I had had quite enough, thank you very much.

Before it was over, I had breakthrough vaginal bleeding, so that meant hormone therapy. Seems every little pore of me was affected by this therapy.

But, you know, that was my price of survival. Without Methotrexate, the transplant would fail; it teaches T-cells to behave so the "Great Immuno-cell War" will not begin.

Leukovorin is the rescue drug that retrieves the white count and tames Methotrexate. Switch-off days of plus-four, seven and thirteen brought almost instant feelings of relative normalcy.

This entire drug switch-off game was my representational leap off the cliff. I had to believe a soft landing was there, waiting for me at the bottom.

By six days post-transplant, eleven days since my journey began, I woke up to find clumps of hair on my pillow. I was becoming bald, and had a heck of a tan. Radiation had given me new moles, and had firmed up my breast tissues; too bad that didn't last. Guess they cooked me enough to get the job done, but not so long as to leave me totally and forever changed physically.

I knew the hair thing was coming, did not know when to expect it though, and was feeling ambivalence around the fact of that loss.

A new adventure was beginning, me bald. I did not want to lose my hair slowly, like a dog with mange. I wanted my hair gone. The reality of my baldness needed to be present, stared in the eye, accepted and appreciated for what it represented.

So, Carol and I planned a clipper party and shaved my head late one afternoon before she left for the day. I sat in the chair in front of my mirror, placed a towel over my shoulders and Carol walked the short distance to the closet to get the clippers. We chatted and laughed as we slowly, methodically, shaved my head one section at a time. The knots and indentations of my skull became apparent. The next reality that crept into my mind: my splotchy, mostly hairless, shiny head immediately became the beacon to others that I was sick and fighting for my life; the signal that my body and soul were changing forever.

With every pass of the clippers over my knotty old head, I realized that my baldness was not bothering me. It was an awakening. I was looking at myself feeling a smile coming. I could live with this, different but tolerable. My past was leaving with each clump of hair on the towel around my shoulders. I believed in my soul; I will survive. I will be new DNA. I will get a new head of hair and a new life. This reality was one of joy.

I had to sleep with a toboggan on my head that night, and every night after; I was cold constantly. You forget why you need hair until it is gone, and it is not to look good. For those of you not from this area of the country, a toboggan or "boggan" is a wool cap we wear on our heads in the winter.

Larry was on sibling duty that week. He came in the next morning carrying a cup of coffee for me, and a paper for him. Odd, but I still wanted and drank coffee; mochas no less. There were so very few foods I even wanted to try; chemo and radiation destroy taste buds and all that was left was the taste of salt. I like salt but not all salt all the time. Coffee covered up the salt, I guess.

That morning, as usual, I was sitting on my bed and my sweatshirt hood was pulled over my head. Larry had also brought a camera with orders from his twin to take pictures. He set the coffee on my tray table and sat down. He then cocked his head to the side and looked at me with a curious look in his blue eyes.

"Why have you got a hood on?"

"Oh, I guess I'm cold. Carol and I cut all my hair off yesterday."

I grinned, but really had a sense of fear of exposure. Larry would be the first person besides my medical team to see my knotty old head.

"Janet, I wish you had waited, I wanted to be here. Let's see."

"Why didn't you tell me you wanted to be here? I would have waited on you."

"It doesn't matter, let's see."

I dropped the hood and struck a pose as Larry laughed and snapped away. Larry stopped the snapping and stared at my bald head and at me for a few moments and a grin slowly elevated the corners of his mouth.

"You know, Sis, doesn't look bad at all."

Larry took a few more shots. I was modeling for the next issue of the bald woman's fashion magazine. This is now the famous Unabomber pose. All I needed was a pair of sunglasses.

After the photo sessions were done, I was sitting on the side of the bed and noticed little red spots all over me.

"Larry, look at this, what do you think?"

"Janet, your platelets are way down. You are bleeding into your skin; Carol is bringing you a platelet transfusion."

"Oh, I knew that." I did not: false bravada.

I realized that little voice of fear had crept into my ear. "No platelets, kiddo, bleeding out?"

The thought of dying hit home with this treatment. My reality: I had no functioning bone marrow. I was really dancing on the ice today. I thought it odd how most days I did real well with my journey and my environment. Then something major would happen and the looming precariousness of my life jumped out of the closet like an ogre in the haunted house at Halloween. And like a child experiencing that moment, I would have that startling scream of total fright, if only in my mind.

I had two platelet transfusions over the next week. Each one meant I was still not making my own. Each transfusion told me the graft was being ignored. My red cell count never dropped below 30 percent so thankfully I didn't need any blood transfused. I believe not becoming anemic (typical for myeloproliferative disease) made me feel stronger than some patients, another blessing.

I chugged along, waiting for that magical and miraculous word, "engraftment." Day 13 came and went. Strangely, I had no fear. It was just another day. I sensed no panic around me from Larry, my nurses, or my doctors.

Becky was not with me; she was far away in Atlanta and she was not so calm. Not being around to see the lack of panic on my end she entered into total fear mode. She called Carey Clifton, one of the stem cell nurse practioners. Becky, in the full throes of her total tears and fear mode, wanted to know why I wasn't engrafting.

Becky the business person and little sister did not understand what was happening or not happening, nor why. Why was I not on schedule? She was so scared and so upset. Becky's tears and her fear told Carey to pass her on to Sharon Sims.

Sharon was my primary nurse practitioner and cool as a cucumber. She looks like and reminds me of Jane Pauley. She listened to Becky's fears, and told her there were other options if I was slow to engraft; I was not that far off of target and to just give my body time. Sharon calmly and firmly told my scared little sister, "Becky, Janet will engraft on her own schedule, not yours."

Becky hung up the phone, feeling somewhat better, but she still wanted me on her schedule. She had that schedule down to the minute.

Sharon came by that afternoon and told me of Becky's fear call. I thanked Sharon for being there for Becky. I knew my little sister would be the impatient one, but that is only because she loves me and needed this phase to end. Really, we all did.

Day 14 post-transplant, Carol came in with my data sheet, as usual. Larry was still there and soon to leave. Becky was next up on the care list. She had scheduled Laura to come in as I was entering the apartment. Jack had a hospital week in there too but was mostly slated for apartment time, as was Mary. Carol handed the sheet to Larry. He grinned and handed it back to Carol.

"What?" I looked at Carol.

Carol grinned as well, and in a whispering voice, almost as if saying the words too loud would pop the news like a bubble,

"Your white count is rising; you are probably engrafted. The doctors will let you know for sure. Do you want to keep this sheet for your memory?"

"Yeah, that would be great."

An inner glow started in the pit of my stomach and rippled to each cell in my body. I had just pulled the ripcord on my freefall off my cliff; the pop jerked me back into the world of possibilities.

I looked at Larry and said, "Let Becky know, please."

Larry left and called everybody.

My sigh of relief at engraftment was short-lived however. I felt like one of Pat Summit's Lady Vol ball players. I was reminded that only this one game was done and won. Another, more difficult game was coming. Keep fighting, keep doing your job of surviving, stay positive, and be gracious under fire. Trust.

I had made it through phase II, one more milestone down, a million to go. Now I had to stay healthy, no GVHD, graft versus host disease, (I had no control over this). No BOOP, bronchiolitis obliterans with organizing pneumonia; a type of immune system attack on the lungs by the donor's cells (no control over this). No CMV, cytomegalo virus, normally seen in childhood respiratory disease. This virus may recurdese when a patient who has been exposed to this virus in the past, is immunosupressed. Blood samples are used to monitor its reactivation. CMV, if it appears, can cause serious gastrointestinal disease or pneumonia (no control over these either). I had to keep the world from reaching into my bubble by not getting an infectious disease like a viral or fungal infection, or a bacterial infection, or a parasite or from other people or inanimate objects around me.

The treatment with methotrexate was finally over. The ulcers in the back of my throat were healing and I could swallow solid food. Tired of popsicles, Maggie Moo milkshakes and of every morsel tasting like salt, real food was calling me, even though it too would taste of salt. Still, hunger was an important step.

Not too much later in the day Mom, Mary and Don came to visit. Another reality came home to roost.

I was fighting so hard to survive; Mom's daily life had been in the back of my mind. I spoke with her every day and I was depending on those around me to take care of her. Mostly I was counting on Mom taking care of herself. She had good health and a strong mind. I thought she would be fine.

This visit showed me I could not depend on any of those thoughts. Mom looked so small, so thin and old. I knew living alone in our big old house was hard for her. She had the dogs to care for and keep her company, but she didn't have anyone to share the day with and isolation is not good for elderly people.

She had lost weight, so I knew she wasn't eating right. Mom is not a fretter but this time the stress of my disease on her life was obvious. I was concerned for her, I knew she was strong, but I also knew she was alone.

Today was a good day for her to have come. She needed to be there on the day the transplant set itself to work. This day gave her more hope that her solitary life had a light at the end of the tunnel.

I spent my remaining hospital time hoping I did not get sick with CMV, praying I did not develop GVHD and that the graft was continuing to take hold.

One of my greatest fears during treatment was the thought of having to take prednisone. I despise the side effects and the lack of life I have with that drug. I prayed a lot over that issue.

The doses would have to be incredibly high if I developed GVHD or BOOP; funny that the fear of taking prednisone had more weight than the transplant.

I suppose it was the difference in what each meant. Transplant was a temporary state; I survived or didn't. Post-transplant is for the rest of my life. I did not like the idea of pred for the rest of my life. The fear was unimaginable. I had to avoid that drug.

CHAPTER THIRTY-SEVEN

"In order to laugh, you must be able to play with your pain."

Annette Goodheart

During my time in the hospital, Social Security had finally sent additional papers to fill out. You guessed it: I had about four days to get them finished and returned to the disability office, which thankfully was located in Nashville. Linda Hudson, the social worker, told me not to worry: "They never turn down an allo."

I started laughing. Linda looked at me with a puzzled look.

"Well, you are looking at one."

"What?"

Linda sat back in her chair.

"They never turn them down; did they really?"

"Yep, they told me I was not sick enough to be disabled." I was still laughing.

"I can't believe that!" was all Linda could say.

Linda took care of the social issues around transplant patients, all the while taking care of her dad who, was also in and out of the transplant ward. Huge hearts were everywhere in this institution.

Becky had called Linda and asked her if she could help fill out the form. By now, cyclosporine had affected my eyes and I could not focus to read the questions. I was shaking so badly I could not write and my ability to mentally focus was poor. I still have memory problems. Thank you for helping me, Linda.

The paper work indicated that their decision would come in 30 to 60 days. I fully expected to be turned down again. So many bad results were storied to have come out of this process. I guess I was gun-shy. I don't know, sometimes it seemed they were waiting to see if I was going to die.

Around 9 o'clock a.m., on my 21st day post-transplant, the door loudly popped open to let my doctors into my world. Dr. Greer finished his physical. He stepped back from the side of my bed, grinned and said those magic words all transplant patients are waiting to hear: "Janet, you can go to the apartment."

"Really? When?"

"Tomorrow after lunch; that should give us enough time to get all the paper work done."

"I have to call Becky! Thanks, Dr. Greer." He smiled and turned and left, knowing for once he had given me good news.

I was ecstatic; if I had had the extra energy I would have done the happy dance. I'm going almost home. I punched in the number and I heard the ring.

"Becky Smith."

"Hey, Sis, I can leave!"

"What! When?"

"Tomorrow afternoon!"

"Thursday! Oh, good grief! Laura doesn't come until Sunday."

(This was another of the periods of time in which I had had to be alone; we weren't counting on me getting out early either.)

"I know, Sis; what can we do?"

"I'll call you back."

Another dilemma to solve; Becky called back in about an hour.

"Sis, I will see you tomorrow afternoon."

My disease had messed up the "schedule" again! I knew Becky had had to make another great sacrifice. Man, was I blessed.

"Be careful, Sis, see you tomorrow."

I had been in my little hospital room for 26 days, four less than expected. I could not wait to leave. My Hickman catheter was still in my chest, and would be for a while longer, but I was free of all the lines, the IV pole, the catheter in my bladder, the morphine for my throat and the subsequent soap capsules that went with it and the uncertainty of engraftment.

I could swallow my medications now, so no more I.V. drugs. Less than a fourth of the way through 100 days and I had hit a major milestone. I started packing with fervor that night. The next morning, the doctors had given the discharge instructions, the prescriptions, and a next appointment time for the clinic. Becky rolled in the door about 2 p.m. She collected my prescriptions and took them to the pharmacy downstairs.

The floor staff helped carry all of my pictures, clothes, music, books and newly acquired hats out to the car. Becky picked up my meds from the pharmacy and paid for $2000 worth of drugs, a month's worth of lifeline.

Leaving the floor, I looked back over my shoulder at the little room where I, with great nurses, doctors, staff and family support, had managed to keep myself together long enough to slay the dragon called transplant.

The nurses smiled, hugged me goodbye and wished me well. Tears of leaving were filling my eyes; I owed them all so very much. Only my living would be payment enough for their compassion and care.

"Come back to see us; we never see our patients after they go home." Louise seemed sad they were a forgotten lot.

The promise was made to come back and see them. The floor staff had become a tightly woven strand in the fabric of my past, a piece of my fabric that would need to be snagged and re-worn occasionally to keep me honest about my future. I resolved to not forget what I had come through, nor to forget those who helped me survive.

My new reality was in focus; only seventy-five more days of fighting this disease in Nashville. I had seventy-five more days of determined, focused behavior to survive, seventy-five more days until I would be going back to my own home and my own room with my mom and my dogs. I had a mere seventy-five more days full of wondering if it would all work. Three months ahead in the apartment, three more months of hospital visits every other day. I could do this. I could see myself on the other side and the view was getting better each day.

Now I continued to hope that BOOP, CMV or GVHD would not show their faces. I continued to pray that I would not pick up a fungal infection or a viral infection. I had missed every bullet so far, described as the poster child for a transplant. I had to stay mobile and one step ahead of the dangers the real world contained. I was ready to go to the next phase of the journey and prepared myself to face the consequences of that phase.

Nonetheless, my ride down the "people" elevator was odd. I was in a wheelchair, was shiny bald, wearing a mask, weak, incredibly tired, toothpick thin, tan and still so close to losing it all. I was one happy little pup! Mary the aide wheeled me through the waiting room where this all began and out the front doors of Vanderbilt Hospital into the wonderful warm sunshine and fall air. Freedom!

CHAPTER THIRTY-EIGHT

"I won't forget this debt, I'm pulling through."
Arthur Herzog and Irene Kitchings

I do not know how to present this in any other way than to tell some stories about the people who took care of me daily or those who never let me forget I was still part of life. Conversations were many: some inane, some mundane, some poignant, but often just small, irrelevant chatter that kept me in the flow of life.

All that I can say is that in my eyes the staff and doctors of VUMC, 11 North, were nothing less than fantastic to me while I lived under their care. Each was knowledgeable, capable, compassionate and most often present.

My nurse practitioners were there every morning before the doctors made their rounds. Early every day, Sharon and Katie were knocking on my door, happy, smiling and ready to answer any questions I might have. There to ask questions of me, to do exams, and to keep the doctors informed and to keep treatment on course.

The nurses were always very aware of each patient's status, the family that was present and the patient's need for encouragement and the occasional reality check. They kept us involved in the day and up to date on our progress toward health.

The staff whose jobs included cleaning, delivering lunch,

making beds, taking vitals: again all wonderful, caring people. It seemed my blessings would not end.

My friends kept me in the world I had left the day Vandy took over my life. Susan and David sent me a video of Topper and Heather. It was a comfort to see they were happy little dogs. Susan was my distant rock; I was blessed to count her a friend then and especially now that my journey has reached this stage of the trip.

One of Becky's routines was to send a daily update to all of my friends. I did not know this but she had requested people send me a hat if they wanted to send me a gift. You cannot receive flowers on the transplant ward: too many soil bad boys. Food was not high on my list of priorities so books and music and hats were very good choices.

One hat in particular was the reason for a lot of laughter among the staff. One day I received a package from Dr. Ann. I opened it up and found the oddest hat I had ever seen. It was made of a heavy multi-colored material with dreadlock-like braids hanging off the edges. The note mentioned that she didn't think Nashville would appreciate the hat but to wear it when I came back to Mobile or New Orleans.

What a hit! Mom wore it but the funniest wearer of the hat was my caretaker, "Dennis, the menace." Dennis was a joy; he kept you laughing and was always smiling and sharing. He found the hat and we put it on his head and we started clowning and taking pictures. What a great release valve.

All of my charge nurses on 11 North were more than excellent; they were top-notch. Teresa, Louise, Carol and Tanya all gave me what I needed in different ways.

Carol was my cheerleader. Never would a day go by that Carol did not remind me that I was going to conquer this disease. Every day,

"You're a survivor, I see it in your face, and you're going to make it."

Carol was there helping me shave my head when hair began to fall out. She talked to me as if I was a valuable human being, with relevant opinions, and she engaged me in conversation to keep me in the daily flow of life outside the transplant ward. Carol was not going to let me focus on the trials of the day; still too much promise in life to spend my day in what-ifs.

Louise was a tall, quiet woman, definitely strong and silent. Her presence was so calming. She was very efficient in her tasks and very open to questions and just a short chat. She kept me peaceful just by walking in the room.

Teresa was so down to earth and easy to deal with during times when I was not so easy. She too was always smiling and doing her job with the seriousness that it required.

Tanya was my night nurse. She was a hoot, always joking and giving me a hard time. Her favorite ribbing of me was centered about one of my wardrobe items.

I wore TED socks every day. They were thigh high socks. One morning, I decided I needed to walk. It was around 3 a.m. and I could not sleep and TV only occupies you so long. You can't leave the unit, so you walk the hall around the nursing stations.

That morning I had on my socks, a T-shirt, and my red running shorts. I had my IV pole, my urine bag, my mask and my shoes. I was styling! Out the door I go. Tanya about ran over me as I exited my room.

"Oh, my gosh!" She could not stop laughing.

"What are you doing?" She was doubled over, tears running down her cheeks.

"You look so stupid. Oh! What a garb." I grinned behind my mask and kept moving.

"You need to sleep. Let me see what is ordered."

Tanya was still laughing. After a couple of rounds by the nursing station I guess Tanya had had enough. She herded me back into my cell and placed me into a state of recumbent stupor. I barely remember taking the Ambien. I slept, deeply, not even remembering Tanya drawing blood about an hour later. Last time I saw Tanya that event was the first question on her lips.

"Why didn't you wear your outfit? I am sure everyone here would love to see it!" I retired that particular look shortly after leaving the hospital.

Tracy was my aide. She took my vitals and changed my bed, and helped with keeping me comfortable. Tall, thin, red-headed, she would spend time talking while she did her job. I have seen her many times since and she is still the same, warm, caring person.

Mary and Dennis were the others who rounded out the people who cared for me. Even the cleaning staff was warm and caring. On a recent visit they gave me my first hugs. Becky was with me; she was crying.

I can never thank Russ Corley enough for his prayerful support. Daily, Russ would come in around 11 in the morning. We would talk about how I was doing and then read a passage from Psalms and say a prayer. Russ was a calming presence during my stay, and kept me closer to God daily.

The doctors were always there, rounds every morning, eight or nine people crammed in that little room full of my stuff. Dr. Greer was an LSU graduate, and I was a Tennessee graduate. I wore a T-shirt that was a banner of achievements that graduates of the University of Tennessee had garnered.

"Janet, what is on that shirt?" he asked one day.

I turned around and let him read it.

"Astronauts, Rhodes Scholars (one of which was Becky's classmate in high school at Rockwood). Somebody reading that shirt would believe that UT is a great academic college. Makes me mad to see UT claiming status as an educational institution."

"Well Doc, the facts speak for themselves." He still grumbled as to the lack of belief in those facts.

Dr. Morgan was a man of "great taste." Tall, thin, blondish, he dressed well, wore an earring in his ear and was nice-looking. He always had a funny comment about something every morning. He'd comment on my pajamas or my food or my bald head, something. One day I had a bowl of brown, gooey food on my table. He stood there looking at it with a slight upturn of his nose.

"What is in that bowl, Janet?"

"Peanut butter and banana."

"Ooh. Wow, really? I haven't had that in years! I ate it all the time as a kid."

I offered him a bite of this culinary delight but he declined. His loss on that one; Larry had made a good batch.

The compassion, care, ability and knowledge never ended during my stay. I am glad I followed my instincts and allowed Vanderbilt to be my transplant site. There is much to be said for the personal touch in medical care. Knowing your doctors and nurses and them knowing you and your family is vital. This was a point that Dr. Wolff had really tried to drive home. He was absolutely correct.

The communities around the hospital contributed to the comfort of transplant patients as well. Massage students came in and gave a free massage; art therapists came and taught patients relaxation techniques, combining them with art. The leukemia society would sponsor lunches.

One particularly bad day, I curled up in bed, needing quiet. My body was so tired and I was so sick. It was about noon. Suddenly, I sat up. There was an eerie calm to the standard noise level of the ward. Then, the most beautiful, ephemeral sound I had ever heard covered my body like a cocoon. Peace. One of the student harpists was sharing her gift with the patients on the transplant ward. Gorgeous. My spirits lifted immediately; I smiled inside. Sleep was easy after that moment.

CHAPTER THIRTY-NINE

"It is well to be up before daybreak, for such habits contribute to health, wealth, and wisdom."

Aristotle

While the mental and emotional experience of leaving the hospital was joyous, my actual entry into the apartment was again anticlimactic. The reality of the disease process had once again pulled me up short. Too weak and tired to much care where I was, the IV pole was still my friend and companion, even here. My magnesium levels would not stay in the proper range because of the cyclosporine, so I had to have infusions twice daily. Initially, home health care nurses took care of this treatment. Becky was with me right after I left the hospital and she had no clue how to hook up an IV line. She didn't want to know.

I did not need the nurse; I could do the treatment myself, but initially, Becky was happier when the nurse came to help. Of course, Larry and Laura could do it. Overall, Jack, Becky and Mary were very pleased they did not need to do this medical "thing."

My day still began early. I was usually up before dawn, said my prayers for the day, would take a shower, walk down the stairs to the couch, turn on the TV and immediately go back to sleep. I was not very hungry, but my caretakers were told to beef me up with protein, protein, protein!

The medical visits were scheduled three times a week. On day 29, I had my next to last bone marrow tap. The DNA was all Laura and still a large amount of scar tissue in the marrow. Several years would pass before all the marrow cavity scarring was expected to be diminished.

Medications did not lessen. I had about eight different medications to take up to twice daily. A closet next to the dining room table held my cache. A list told me what to take when. How I kept them straight at first, I do not know. In time, it was second nature and Becky bought a pill holder that would cover an entire day and all week.

My goal: exercise more every day as I got stronger. The Vanderbilt campus is beautiful any time of year. The trees and grounds are unique, the sculpture throughout the campus is thought-provoking, and the chimes are peaceful. As the day warmed, whoever was with me would take me out onto the campus. Each day I could go farther.

One day, I wanted to go into Hillsboro village at the foot of the hill below the apartment. Hillsboro is a quaint area with restaurants and shops. Home of the famous Pancake Pantry, which was always so full I never got to eat there, art stores, book stores, craft stores, clothes, food, whatever you could want to buy was available somewhere in Hillsboro village.

I had forgotten the walk would be a climb up and then down and coming home a huge climb up. I just wanted out of my cage for a while. Mary and I started chatting and laughing as we got in the elevator to take us down to 21st street. About halfway up the first hill, in front of Peabody College, I knew I was pushing my luck.

"Janet, are you sure you are going to be able to do this?"

I was weak, and having difficulty breathing. Lying in a bed for 30-plus days destroys your ability to easily use muscles.

They do not exist anymore, really; if you don't use it you lose it. I had tried to exercise while in the hospital; it was never enough to overcome the disease and the treatment. So, I put on my stubborn, determined-to-win-this-one Smith mask and replied, "Yes, I will be fine, just let me sit down a second."

The traffic on the street was sending huge clouds of nauseating gases in my direction.

"OK, if you are sure. We can go back. Or I can go and get the car and we will just drive down."

"No, I can do it. Driving won't meet the goal."

I managed and learned that if I was going to do anything physical there had to be a plan and I must save energy. The price was exacted on both the physical scale, if too much was attempted, and the emotional scale if the goal attempted was not met.

Shortly after entering the apartment, a letter arrived from the Social Security Administration. Honestly, the whole Social Security charade had moved off my radar screen so the letter was another snap back into the real world. I was alive and needed to pay my bills. I shook my head as I tore open the letter, wondering what new insight into me the SSA would have this time. Before reading it, I checked the letter date and the postmark. Yep, five-day difference; with delivery time seven days consumed. I began to read the letter.

SSA has decided: on second analysis you meet the definition of disabled (Surprise! since August) and your benefits scheduled to begin six months from the time we declared you as disabled. So almost one year after applying, I would finally receive some income.

BC/BS, under the transplant contract, would reimburse living expenses incurred during my stay in Nashville at 80 percent. Becky had taken on the payment of these outside expenses. She paid for the apartment and my first round of meds. I am grateful she would regain most of her monies. I had supplemental insurance with Physician's Mutual Insurance. These policies were very helpful in that they paid me, not the hospital. The cash was so very much needed and I am glad I chose to add them as a supplement years before becoming ill.

Traffic into and out of the apartment was pretty limited by design. My cousins came, a few friends that just happened to be in Nashville came, but mostly it was just us.

Again, the family had to take care of their own lives to help me take care of mine. So, soon they all learned they could leave me alone for a while at a time; I wasn't going to break. Larry started touring Nashville, attending lectures at Vanderbilt, drawing birds, going to country music clubs and visiting family. He kept trying to get me to go with him. What was he thinking?

Jack found he could play golf and spend time with his friends. There were no phones ringing or email to deal with, just quiet and time to relax, a rare occurrence in his life. He enjoyed the quiet and read a lot. The girls exercised, shopped, visited with family, read and had a good time.

Their temporary absence was just what I needed! I loved that they were there but everybody needs some down time away from others so to recharge. My definition of recharge was sleep.

The Vanderbilt school was next door to the apartment and watching the kids play at recess brought joyous memories of my past. The laughter and physical-ness of kids at play gave me hope. Every morning they would be dropped off by their parents and they would wander through the gates, two by two into their classrooms. All in brightly-colored clothing with backpacks bigger than they were. It brought back memories of me at their age. The joy they found in simple things, boundless energy, never a thought of mortality: just thoughts of the day and the promise of a great future.

I needed God's other creatures around as well so I put food out on the porch at the apartment for the birds and the squirrels. I could sit on the couch and watch them fill their crops or their bellies.

Mom visited me at the apartment a time or two but the trip was long and she didn't come often. Don and Mary were so good to her while I was sick. They took that worry off my plate to some degree. Every day I would call her and check in with progress reports and queries as to her health. Our neighbors would call and check in on her.

Sara Mee, our neighbor of 40 years, told me after I came home that during my time away Mom would never ask for anything and just kept saying she would be fine when Janet got home and that "so far" everything was going okay. Seems we all waited for that other shoe to drop.

Becky's watch included Thanksgiving. We called several times, trying to get Mom to come up but she did not want to leave home. Becky loves Thanksgiving; it is her holiday. This would be her first not spent with Mom and at home. She was very sad and a little put out with Mom for not letting her come to get her. Mom had her Thanksgiving in Rockwood with Mary and Don.

Becky and I decided to go into downtown Nashville and have our Thanksgiving dinner. I sure looked odd in that nice restaurant with my mask covered face and my bandana covering my bald head with a hat perched on top. People stared at my thin, sick body covered in gray flannel slacks that just did not fit anymore. Who cared? I was alive and having Thanksgiving dinner with my little sister.

Never mind the food still tasted like salt. The turkey looked good on the plate, and Becky said it was all quite tasty, especially the pumpkin bisque, smooth and sweet yet with a quick bite left behind on the tongue. Best meal I had ever eaten!

Most importantly, I was present. The day was warm and sunny, downtown was quiet. I did not need to taste my Thanksgiving Day meal. I trusted Becky that the food was good and imagined the taste of each morsel. The overriding lesson of the day: Life is good. Truly, a blessing to be thankful for on that day designed for giving thanks.

The passing days helped me reach the stage in my recovery where I could go out more often. Mary and I would go to the hospital, and when my visit was over we would go out to eat lunch. We always sat away from the crowd and chose off-hours to eat. This protected me from exposure to other's illnesses. I had to eat only well-cooked food, no fresh vegetables or fruits. I asked but Dr. Kassim would not let me eat sushi yet. He just could not understand why I would want to.

Other aspects of living had regulations as well. The nurses were there to remind me that sex was out of the question. Funny, that somehow was not on my agenda. I could barely walk across the room.

"Not a problem!" was all I said.

My 100 days was finally close to an end. I had taken care of myself, had washed my hands obsessively, had worn my mask obsessively, and tried not to expose myself to disease. I had not developed BOOP, CMV or GVHD and thus missed the prednisone bullet! I had escaped the trap. December had arrived. I had had a bubble around me for the last four months. Christmas was coming; I wanted out of Nashville.

For the first time since beginning this journey, my self-descriptive included agitated and depressed. Emotions dictated; move on, now! Ready to go home, I did what all self-respecting people who are dependent upon the will of others do. I begged; shamelessly, boldly and constantly.

Poor Dr. Kassim was the victim who was to fall prey to this mantra at one of my weekly visits. We had finished my exam and were just chatting about stuff when I brought up the option.

"Dr. Kassim, please, let me go home. I am doing better, not sick, and can get back here within two hours if I need to. Christmas is coming and I want to go home. I miss my dogs, my friends and my own bed."

He sat quietly, starting with a grin, then a head shaking. "No, you need to stay here the 90 days per post-transplant protocol."

This prompted Mary and she chimed in right behind me, adding more fuel to this bonfire of shamelessness. I did not know we could be so whiny!

"Oh, yes, please let her go. It is almost Christmas. What a great gift. Ninety days is nearly gone anyway. Please."

By Dec. 12, almost three months since leaving the hospital, came the words I wanted to hear. Doc's warm, jovial, round face gave form to a big smile and with a nod of his head he said,

"OK, Janet, you can go, but no sushi!"

"Sounds just fine to me, Doc. Not a problem."

The trip back to the apartment that morning took an eternity. I had to pack and get out of there! Those four walls that had once been my salvation were now morphing into a new kind of jail. I needed that commuted sentence and the freedom to go home and I got it.

We had slowly taken most of my cursory items home. Clothes and food were the only things left. It was the middle of the month and we had paid rent for the entire month. We could come back later and finish clearing it out.

Mary and I loaded up the car, piled in and drove home in the rain. Tears of joy for me, I was going home. The long drive along I-40 E was a reversing of my trip into the unknown, and the goal now was to stay home and finish healing. Before we left Nashville we called Don and I told him not to tell Mom I was coming home.

Three hours later, Mary and I pulled into the driveway. I was so excited that I nearly leaped out of the car. I stood at the door and rang the bell. The dogs barked the alarm. I stepped away from the door, down the stairs and to the side of the house. Mom opened the door looked around, saw no one and wondered who had gotten her out of her chair. I popped around the corner.

"Hi, Mom

She stepped back, that beautiful smile of hers all over her face.

"You get in here!"

We grabbed each other and hugged a long time. Topper and Heather were at my feet crying for attention. I was so happy to be home.

Walking into my bedroom, looking at the picture of my dad hanging on the wall, I sat on the edge of my bed and tears finally fell. I had made it down the river Styx with all its precariousness. I was home. The tears were short lived and replaced with laughter and joy.

CHAPTER FORTY

"Janet, we will see you in January 2002 "

One hundred days completed; time for "the milestone" exam. I was dreading the full two days of testing looming before me. Some of these tests would be painful, some of them long, all of them telling of my future. There were appointments with pulmonologists to make sure I was not developing BOOP (using radiographs, CT's and pulmonary function tests), dermatologists would take skin biopsies to make sure I was not developing GVHD, nuclear medicine people would do a MUGA scan to make sure my heart had not been damaged by the chemotherapy and radiation therapy, ophthalmologists would check my tear production for dry eye and make sure no cataracts were forming.

Finally, Madan would pull blood and perform one more bone marrow tap. Hopefully the Hickman catheter, a constant in my life since September 2001, could be removed from my chest. This bone marrow tap was my last tap, providing my transplant held. Dr. Madan had said up front that if the transplant held less than 18 months I could not be re-transplanted.

A much harried, busy, young surgery resident; with some prodding from Madan, finally removed the Hickman from my chest late the second evening. Becky and I did not get home until very late. Who cares, my last vestige of transplant was gone!

A few weeks later and the results came in: dry eye, but all other tests were in line, all donor DNA and, as expected my marrow cavity was still scarred.

The six-month post-transplant mark meant my medicine load could start to decrease. Drug costs were going to drop. My eyes would focus and the shaking would disappear. The antibiotics and the anti-fungals, and the immunosuppressants, and the anti-depressants would soon be unnecessary. Seeing a light at the end of the tunnel my focus narrowed and my pace increased as I ran straight to that light of a life to be regained.

My body was stronger. I took a nap every day, sometimes twice a day. My taste buds were slowly returning to normal. Hair was starting to grow and it had totally changed character. Born with thin, straight, blondish brown hair; it was growing back as thick, curly, dark hair instead. I prayed it would revert to type but the important fact, I reminded myself, was that in this moment I was growing hair and eyelashes.

My body had physically changed: very thin and getting thinner. My muscle mass had dropped and my shape changed. An athlete all of my life, playing basketball, being a lifeguard, jumping horses, water skiing, lifting weights, running; I enjoyed being active. Built like a swimmer, with broad shoulders, thin hips and long legs, my new image was morphing into a stick. Shoulders were bony, my hips non-existent, and my long legs were so skinny I was knobby. I wanted to start getting physical to try to regain some muscle and strength.

Working in the yard is one of my passions. I love the physicalness of digging and planting and mulching and watching my work add texture and color to the yard. By March, seven months post-transplant, the weather was warming and I was decreasing my dose of Cyclosporine. I put on my mask and started to work. At first 15 minutes, then 45 and reaching one hour was a major accomplishment. Never mind I used to be able to work hard all day, only stopping to eat lunch. I was so excited to be doing anything that smacked of normal. My life was going to be regained; I felt it.

Follow-up trips to Vandy came about every month. Becky, Jack, Mary and Don all took turns driving me out to Nashville. They decided that I was still too sick to do the trip alone. I knew better than to try to fight this notion. The point being, my family gave up huge chunks of their time and lives for me during my ordeal. My cup had overflowed and appeared bottomless. God's grace was boundless in my life.

Nothing but clear sailing; all the clichés you can muster were present on the tip of my tongue. I had made it!

CHAPTER FORTY-ONE

"A stitch in time saves nine."

By June 2002, less than one year past my transplant, less than two months off cyclosporine, I noticed I was having difficulty breathing when I exercised. I thought it was just my body learning to work again. In true Janet fashion, I ignored it.

By July, my family had noticed I could not talk without being winded. By August, I could not breathe very well at all. While communicating with Dr. Madan he told me to have a lung CT pronto. We were concerned I might be developing BOOP. Dr.Dobbs' office set up the lung CT at Baptist in Knoxville. The radiologist from Baptist would fax the result of the CT to Madan that afternoon.

I called Dr. J. and the nurse at Vandy told me they had not received the information. Baptist said they sent it. Calling Vandy back later that afternoon, she said they would check. I did not hear an answer that evening.

News travels fast in this clan. Becky had called me around 8:30 and was not happy with my state of affairs. Becky called Larry. Larry called me around 9 p.m. He was coaching his son's football team and had to step away from the action to call.

"Janet, Becky says you can't even talk."

Uh-oh, his "I am a concerned brother who is in that doctor mode" again. I wanted to hang up! He would have called me right back so why bother?

"Well… I think… that that… is just… a little ex… ag…ger…ated." Pushing air and trying to hold a convincing conversation with a doctor on the other end of the line was becoming a joke.

"Doesn't sound like it. What are you doing about this?"

"I had… a CT… done at Bap…tist… and they… are… to send the results… to Madan."

"Have you heard from him?"

"No, I called… today trying… to find out… if Baptist … had sent… the results… and they said… that they did. Vandy… says they didn't."

"Give me the number out there, this is ridiculous. I'm going to call out there and find out what is going on. Sis, you can't breathe!"

I gave Larry the number, wondering if I really should have let him fight this battle but he was adamant. In 15 minutes, he called back.

"That guy I talked to doesn't know anything about your case. It's a fellow; they never know what is going on. What is Baptist's number?"

"I don't know, ask 411."

"I'll call back in a while."

"Fine."

I had just sat down. The phone rang. I stood and dragged myself across the den and picked up the receiver expecting to hear the voice of another sibling.

"Hello."

"Janet, Madan. What is going on?" Finally! My protector from the horde arrived.

"Larry … wants to know… why the results… aren't in. I called… Baptist today… and they said… they faxed you… the results." I just could not get those words out.

"Janet, I did not get them on my desk. I'll get to the bottom of this and get back with you. I'll call Knoxville now."

"Thanks, Madan."

In about an hour Madan called back with my marching orders: come to the hospital and check in on Tuesday. I asked him to please call Larry. He was more than happy to do so.

In about an hour the phone rang again.

"Hello."

"Sis, I'm sorry I stirred the hornets nest. I talked to Madan."

"Not… a problem… I'm glad… you care enough… to act. Talk soon. I love you."

"Love you too. Goodnight."

The episode was not unnoticed at Vanderbilt. The next morning Madan called. He had tried to keep me out until Tuesday. It was Labor Day weekend. No testing would be done over the holiday. The hospital only had holiday staff. Besides, what was another day or two after dealing with this anomaly for the last few months? Unfortunately for me, Madan did not manage to convince the powers that be and they demanded that I admit through the emergency room on Saturday.

I did not get there until late Saturday night. I told Becky I would drive myself. She was incensed. Coming home for the holiday anyway, she would drive me there and then bring Mom home on her way back to Atlanta. Becky had to drive three-and-a-half hours from Atlanta, pick me up and turn right around and drive two-and-a-half more to Nashville. That is no small feat for Becky; she has back problems that make car travel difficult at best, but the option of me driving myself was squelched early.

The ER at Vandy that night was full of sick, not just injured, people. Becky walked up to the desk and told the receptionist I was there to enter the hospital.

"Have a seat in the waiting room and we will get to you as soon as possible." The receptionist looked at Becky. Becky did not move. I started walking away.

"Janet, don't go in there! It is full of sick people." The BLT had spoken. She turned to the receptionist: "No, she cannot sit in there with all those sick people. She is a transplant patient. She cannot get sick!" The security guard started listening to the conversation.

The receptionist agreed and told her to sit me next to the wall. In a moment, someone from upstairs had come to roll me to my new room on 11 North.

My doctor ordered a bronchoscopy, but no staff was there to do the procedure over the holiday. I lay in the hospital bed for three days receiving breathing treatments and waiting. I was not happy; it seems my tolerance for things medical was not so present this time. This disease had once again parlayed itself into my future. I was becoming well fed up with this lifestyle. A nurse I did not recognize from round one led me into room 11024 this time, Rick's room.

Rick had gotten out of the hospital shortly after I did. He was having some problems with GVHD but had gotten to go to the apartment. Shortly after leaving the hospital, he developed CMV. He had to be readmitted off and on for several months. Eventually Rick developed encephalitis and died before his 100 days were done. There, but for the grace of God go I.

Because of our linked history, Rick's room gave me the creeps. My mind's eye kept seeing him when we were having our transplants, wondering how he felt, how he was dealing with his own family's lack of support. Every day his son was with him watching TV in the dark, blinds closed. Sheri was trying with all she had to get him through this and home. He was all she had; my heart sank when Carol told me Rick had died.

Rick and I spoke briefly to say hello, how ya doing. I would wave as I walked past his door on my morning hall walks. We ordered our milkshakes together. The experience between us did not need words. A look in the hall waiting for our turn in the oven was enough to know a kindred spirit. Rick fought the good fight. I often wonder how Sheri and her son are getting along. I pray God's grace found them a way.

CHAPTER FORTY-TWO

"Only a physician who believes in a potential power for healing that exists within his patient can treat his patient…In a sense the physician can be only the assistant to this power…."

Earl A. Loomis

Early Sunday morning Becky and Mom were visiting me before heading back to East Tennessee. They brought a cup of Starbucks coffee, a sweet roll and the *New York Times*. I was working the puzzle when the door opened to find a very animated, communicative, dark-haired foreign doctor coming into the room. He introduced himself in a European accent as the doctor who had spoken with Larry the fateful night of the CT scan. Very upset about how the situation had transpired, he could not understand why Larry, a doctor himself, had responded to his fellow doctors the way he had. He apologized for any bad feelings that may have arisen, talked about his idea of what was wrong and left.

I never saw him again. I could have told him Larry had apologized for his behavior. I didn't. I wanted the young doctor to realize that siblings get fearful and angry when there is a threat of loss or an appearance of inactivity. It wasn't Larry the doctor he talked to, it was the Larry who knew the medical ropes and "the brother." Madan understood that, had tried to explain to the young doctor and personally let it slide.

The rest of the "doctor teams" came by that morning:

oncologist, infectious disease, pulmonologists and respiratory therapists, blood work teams, on and on. Tuesday morning arrived and testing was in motion. The familiar knock of a year ago came early.

"Ms. Smith?"

"Yes, I'm here, just a minute."

I finished brushing my teeth and opened the door. My chariot awaited me on the other side. I sat down and was off. This time my route was different. I was not immunosupressed so I rode down the regular patient elevator to floor seven. My driver wheeled me into the bronchoscopy room.

"Here's Ms. Smith."

"Fine, thanks."

I saw a thin male doctor, a European from his accent, sitting at the computer screen at the back of the room. The tech helped me out of my chair.

"We need you here on this bed. I will raise the head of it and place this mask on your face. I need to start your lidocaine inhalant."

The process of inhaling lidocaine was messy and it sputtered and spattered into my eyes, burned them and made me nauseous.

Sedation was kicking in; I did not know much else until it was over and I was in my room. I hoped taking samples of my lung tissues would tell my doctors what they needed to know. Biopsy results are only as good as the sample. I was getting tired of this merry-go round, having already grabbed my brass ring a year ago. How many rings were there for one person?

Two days later and the results: inconclusive, not enough tissue to make a diagnosis. We need a whole lung biopsy.

Well, wasn't I excited!

Late Wednesday afternoon the surgeon came by my room to meet me. He was a tall thin dark-headed man of foreign descent. I mention this only to paint a picture. I could care less about the race, religion or nationality of those who took care of me. They just needed to be competent people. This tall, "swarthy man" would put holes in my chest wall, take a piece of my lung, and put air where it didn't belong. He needed to be competent. He introduced himself, I don't remember his name. I do remember his behavior during that meeting.

About three feet from the foot of my bed, he stood there very stiffly with his arms behind him; his white coat was very starched and he never even cracked a smile. The respiratory assistant sat at the foot of my bed.

In a deep foreign accent I heard, "I will not shake your hand." The respiratory aide just dropped his head and I saw a grin forming beneath his nose.

I guess I recoiled. I don't know. All I could think was, how odd. Did I offer my hand? No.

His approach to patient confidence building seemed a little different and the whole scene was funny to me. Not laughing out loud in response during our meeting was difficult. I was so tired any little thing was turning my giggle box and it was hard not to react at times.

"Sure, no big deal." was about the best I could muster.

Was he afraid I had the grip of Wonder Woman and would crush his little hand, or was he afraid that he might give me something deadly? Having a surgeon in our family, I would say it was the former and not the latter. He was protecting himself, I think. We talked about the procedure, a thorascopic biopsy and he left.

Then I started a tearful laughing; I needed that. I was just happy I had kept my composure while he was in the room. I do get silly when I am tired and I did not want to hurt his feelings or anything before he picked up a scalpel.

Sleep that night was poor; I awoke several times. My pulse-ox readings kept dropping and I had to have oxygen therapy and inhalation treatments to breathe. Being awake most of the night led to conversations with the staff.

Knowledge in hospitals travels quickly through the grapevine. That night, while talking to my nurse, I learned that my "swarthy man" surgeon was one of the best and one of Madan's friends, to boot. At the end of it all, the grapevine chatter had convinced me of my safety. I finally slept in peace at the thought of this "swarthy man" who would not shake my un-offered hand, chunking up my lung first thing in the morning.

The afternoon of the biopsy I awoke to find I had three holes in my chest, a quarter-inch diameter plastic chest tube coming out of my right chest wall and bruises on my wrists from getting arterial blood samples. They will heal. I hoped this time they sliced out what they needed.

My chest gave me thought though. Painful, hard to move and, again, I was not so gracious. By Friday, still no answers. Stuck in bed with that tube, I was becoming surlier by the minute. I wanted this over and me home. I was to have the chest tube pulled when the air in my chest, technically a surgically induced pneumothorax, had dissipated to near nothing. Another weekend in the hospital; they expected at least three days post-op before the tube could be yanked.

Monday, radiographic films indicated the air was gone from around my lungs. The tube was pulled. The initial read seemed to indicate either immune mediated or inflammatory. I was hoping for something simple like infectious, treatable with pills. But the doctors were unsure whether the cause was a hypersensitivity reaction to something in my environment, or a GVHD/donor response, BOOP, or Sarcoidosis.

Regardless of the call, each disease process on the

differential list meant steroids. My good buddy prednisone; I bucked. Steroids really make my life hell. I have severe reactions. I can't sleep, I don't eat, I drink too much water, I urinate too much, I get manic, cannot complete anything, I swell like a balloon full of air and I get quite angry and agitated. I do this even at low doses. Even my mom hates me on this drug. That says something about why I hate prednisone.

Mission: do anything to stay off that particular drug.

I asked the lung doctor if she could try inhalant steroids first. Her initial reaction left me holding what breath I had.

"Janet, historically they won't do what we need to do here; I guess we can try. I understand your reluctance to get into a steroid dependency with this disease. Sure, we'll try."

"Thank you, Doc. I will do whatever you say except I will fight you on that drug." I exhaled and took in a breath of victory. At least I thought it was victory.

She laughed and before she left my room she stopped and turned to me.

"Janet, you may want to find a pulmonologist in Knoxville in case there is an emergency. There is a doctor that practices at UT. He completed a residency here and is a very good doctor. His name is Dr. Broncha."

Her recommendation caught me off guard and I burst out laughing. She looked at me with a clueless, stunned look and with an offended tone she spoke. "Why are you laughing?" Her colleague also seemed stunned.

"Well, don't you think that's funny? A pulmonologist named Broncha?"

She still seemed clueless; I let it go.

The final biopsy results had not been completed by Wednesday. Poor Dr. Kassim, I pushed him to his maximum level of patience over this pred issue. He did not yet know of my agreement with the pulmonologists and they were present during this session.

I really like Dr. Kassim, a whole lot; he's funny and warm and we had had many laughs over the course of my disease. He had to listen to me beg to go home early from the transplant. Now he had to listen to this too. Bless his little heart.

He looked tired, was pouting and seemed very put out this time. I realized I was making his life hard and backed off.

"I apologize, but I am not going to take pred without trying something else first. Sorry, that's how I feel."

The tension broken, Dr. Kassim smiled his big face-filling smile then and said we would try first without the steroids. I re-started Cyclosporine, and a new drug called Cellcept. Advair inhaler has a steroid component and they gave me that as well.

Then, heaping insult upon injury—you would think I would know when to hush—I begged Dr. Kassim to let me go home. He sighed and dropped his head, a small grin still lingering on his face. "No, Janet. I want you to stay in hospital until Friday because the lab results should be back by then. We need to know if we need to change your meds."

I reminded him that I was taking a bed that someone sicker than me might need. I begged and pleaded; an unwelcome de'ja' vu for Dr. Kassim since it was less than a year since the last "I want to go home" begging session.

He relented; they would let me go home with my cousin Nancy, who lives in Franklin. She would get me to Vandy on Friday for the results appointment with Madan and Mary and Don would pick me up and bring me home.

Later that evening, before Nancy got to the hospital, Sharon came by my room to see if Dr. Kassim had told me any results.

"No, haven't heard from him."

"Oh, well, I understand that."

Sharon then quietly confided in me. "Janet, you do know too much sometimes. It does make it hard when you know side effects."

I was not sure if Sharon was chastising me or just stating a fact. I responded the way I thought she meant it. "True words, but I was wrong and needed to back off. Dr. Kassim was there to help."

I left with Nancy that evening, glad to be in the September air. Nancy, Gary and I had dinner, looked through old family photos, cried some and went to bed.

Two days passed and on Friday I was traveling back to Vandy to see Madan and get the final biopsy results and any medication changes. The choice was one I did not want to hear, and would not accept as fact.

"Janet, the final biopsy report supported a hypersensitivity reaction. Continue on the medication as planned, you know you're going to have to take steroids with this problem."

"Well, we'll see."

Jagasia scheduled a recheck for three months out.

"Hey, Dr. Madan, the pulmonologists recommended I get a pulmonologist in Knoxville. He did a residency here. His name is Broncha."

Madan about fell out of his chair laughing; I knew he'd get it!

After a month on the protocol, not much was clearing. I called Madan and we decided to try a Medrol pack. He was so patient with my little fear game. It helped; big surprise. After it had left my system, I got worse again. I gave in and started a round of pred, three months' worth of mania. Oh, joy.

CHAPTER FORTY-THREE

"Make the most of yourself, for that is all there is of you."

R.W. Emerson

That fall was such a period of madness and inability to really finish anything. I could not sit still. I audited an art class and was very prolific in my work. I baked and cooked all the time, not wanting to eat it, giving everything away. By the first of the year, the dose of prednisone was to start tapering to the lower end of the dose range. I could not wait. I was exhausted from dealing with my captor and his demands.

By April, one year after the first episode began; I was back to square one. Off drugs once again, and trying to recover my life. That life had to include practicing veterinary medicine again. I had to try to replace my old life by fusing it with the new.

Dr. Dummer, the infectious disease doctor at Vanderbilt, and I met before the transplant to talk about future concerns around my ability to safely practice veterinary medicine. He recommended I not go back to clinical practice anymore, feeling a white-collar job would be best. His concern was based in my loss of immunity to public disease like measles, mumps, flu and others because of the transplant and the drugs I would be taking would only make me more susceptible when exposed.

Dummer was concerned that even after a year off the immunosuppressants I would not be able to have the vaccination for rabies. There was no data on post-transplant vaccination with a rabies vaccine. There was no way to know my body would mount an appropriate response, especially after being on the immunosuppressants. He was concerned that if bitten by a rabid animal, I could not take the treatment without contracting the disease. The damned if you do, damned if you don't routine seemed to apply. I was hoping we could find the answer to this dilemma and it would be in my favor.

Another big issue was my splenectomy. If bitten by an animal, I would have a 60 percent greater risk of becoming septic, i.e., developing a blood infection. There was data to support this conclusion and it seemed that every veterinary conference I attended was driving home the point to spleenless vets. I was much more susceptible to pneumococcus pneumonia and haemophilus influenza.

It did not matter; practicing medicine was my life and I wanted it back. I could be very cautious. Companion animal practice rarely sees rabid animals. If there were any questions, a vaccinated vet could handle that case. Better animal handling and the use of muzzles on aggressive animals would reduce my risk of a bite. If the exam room was full of snarking kids, someone else could go in or bring the animal out. There was a way; I would find that way at the correct time.

Not knowing how my body would respond to being on my feet for long hours while working, I was offering to volunteer at the clinic I had worked in before the transplant. I thought that would be a good environment to try my abilities again; they knew what I had lived through the past couple of years.

The offer would receive a rousing "Oh, yeah, I want you back" routine from my previous clinic. Problem was, every time I tried to set up a time, there was always a reason it wasn't a good time to do it.

I have always been sensitive to the responses, body language and voices of other people. I kept asking myself why my former boss was acting this way. To me it was a simple issue. If the job would not be made available again, why not just tell me? Don't play stupid games; just clear the path one way or another.

My nature drives me to truth. I so much prefer honesty to games. It would not have made a tinker's damn to me if I went back to that job. Just let me know so to put it all behind me and find a new road. The way this issue was handled made me realize my feelings were not important.

The reality: apparent concern shown for my future appeared to have been mostly false. There were always the questions from them wanting to know all about how I was feeling, how was I coping. I became leery of both the true aim of the concern and the entire situation. A straight answer about the clinic position I was told would be waiting for me after the journey was not forthcoming. My heart said, "Let it go for now, give yourself more time and see how the road bends around this issue."

That reality left me needing to exert some other type of positive choice so to regain my past activities in some other realm. Simple, ask Dr. Madan if I could try to start riding horses again; reasonable request from an eager patient trying to regain life.

I called Dr. Madan. Once I heard his voice on the line, I was sure all would be well. Guess I misread that one too! Soon all I heard was the echoing voice of a stunned man that could be heard over the phone line all the way into East Tennessee. Like Cis's farm call, it was ringing into my core as well as my ear.

"*No*, you cannot hang out in a barn right now! There are too many risks from the hay and dirt and manure found in a barn."

He appeared adamant, entrenched and unmovable on this point. Well, I knew what had worked with Kassim. I was not sure the tactic would work with Jagasia. Never know until you try.

Behaving as a whiney child held no shame for me now. I was as a child needing permission to restart my life. The last few years my medical needs and the wants of others directed my activity. I had fallen into that mode of permission-seeking before acting, forgetting the adage of acting, then apologizing later, if needed.

"What if I wear a mask and the trainer brushes and saddles the horse. How can exercise and fresh air be bad for me? I would stay out of the barn and only be outside in the arena."

Again, my passion was talking, not sense. After a few no's from him, followed by a few more "reasonable justifications" from me, Jagasia gave up the fight; he knew I would probably do it anyway. I only carried 125 pounds on a 5'10" frame that had no strong muscle. Exercise found me still breathing hard but I was determined to try to ride again. My soul needed it in the worst way.

Melissa Roberts and her family own Runaway Farms. They breed and train sport ponies. She was happy to help me get back on a horse. Horse people feel there is no life unless you are on or near a horse. The restrictions I had around grooming and the barn were discussed and she was more than happy to get the horse ready. That morning she had Sophie all saddled and ready to go.

I walked the horse into the arena, hopped into the saddle and tried to remember how to ride. My mind knew, but my body had lost all memory. We started at a walk; toward the end of the lesson Melissa asked if I wanted to trot. I did and managed to trot a 20-meter circle. I was so excited and beside myself with glee. I had believed I would never ride again. I felt so alive! I had done it and I continued to ride once a week. Around August, there was a new onset of weakness and difficulty in breathing, a vasculitis and again a low-grade temperature elevation, so back to Vanderbilt.

CT's, lung function tests, skin biopsy and another pulmonologist, Aaron Milstone. I found him a nice man, very bright, and a very good doctor. There was something, though, that I knew would cause us problems in the long run, even though I could not put my finger on it at first. For some reason I always felt on the defensive when in his presence; maybe it was an ego deal (mine or his or both) or maybe his bedside manner. I don't know, may never know why I had that reaction when I had an appointment with his clinic. Regardless of the cause, it made it likely we would butt heads and we did, more than once. Usually every time we met.

This doc doesn't like to lose. He and Dr. Madan have that in common. That's fine; I don't like to lose medically either. But there was something in me that went on guard. Less than a year since being in the hospital for biopsies Milstone wanted another bronchoscopy.

Here we go again. Not in the mood to go back in the hospital for those lung tests, I put on my surly face and got a little assertive. Becoming assertive was not a hard position for me to achieve at this moment of the journey. I was really tired of this play and wanted off the stage.

Sometimes I felt Milstone was not listening to me. I appreciated his talents and experience and his need for testing. On the other hand I felt I had to explain my reluctance to his request.

My flaw of shooting myself in the foot and not separating what I know from the situation was just as present. I was tired, no, exhausted, and becoming more so with every day. This was a certain sign that I had nearly hit the wall with this entire sick business. I remembered how I felt before my initial diagnosis. I felt like a wild animal in a cage, pacing, looking for a way out of my captivity. Given an opportunity, with no one or nothing in particular to attack, I realized I would fight my way out by attacking the whole situation and everyone that got in the scatter range. How easily I had forgotten about my little scene with Kassim a few months before. So the games began.

"Dr. Milstone, the last group of pulmonologists in this building told me they would not base a diagnosis on just a bronchoscopic biopsy, not enough tissue. That happened while I was hospitalized. If the plan today is to do a bronchoscopic biopsy and then follow with a full lung, then just do the lung and don't waste my money."

I was not being stubborn about his desires; only that after two years of medical treatment I also had great concern about my health insurance limits, all of these hospitalizations and tests. These were the other primary issues driving my behavior. I should have told him that up front in a better way. I could not afford to lose my coverage. Being honest around that issue might have helped but this was one rapid-fire conversation without much time to interject real fears and concerns. His agenda was going to go forward. I had thrown a gauntlet and he did not back down from the duel.

"Well, I can make a diagnosis off of the biopsy; I do it all the time. Some of my patients have it done every six months. I have no plan to take another piece of your lung."

"I'm serious about this, Doc; do one or the other, not both. Take your best shot now."

"I can do it with a biopsy."

"Fine, do it then."

Feeling like we had just played a round of "Name that Test," I relaxed at that thought of no thoracoscopy and prayed he was as good as he said he was with a biopsy sample tip.

I was so tired of being poked and cut and prodded and stitched and held captive to drugs and hospitals and the inability to breathe. I was just damn tired and getting angry at my lack of progress through this disease. I felt helpless. I hate helpless.

A week later Mary and Don drove me to Vanderbilt, waited for me to get through the outpatient procedure and wake up. They drove me home while I was still in a semi-drugged state.

Results again indicated a hypersensitivity-induced inflammation of my lungs. Milstone had done blood work looking for any reactant that would explain the problem.

I had called Madan to check on any results; he told me to contact Milstone; there might be an environmental issue here. So, I called Milstone.

"Test the house, Janet. Your mold titer is high. I usually use a company here in Nashville. I am not sure they come into your area. Here is the number."

"OK, I'll call, thanks."

I was stunned and still frustrated, bordering on angry. I hung up and called Becky.

"Sis, they say my lungs are bad because of the house, mold."

Becky was furious. She had to deal with these environmental issues all the time in her work and knew what it would mean to the family if that were true. Becky said she fussed at God, asking why the house?

"She has fought a good fight don't make her leave her home." There was no answer until a few weeks later, after the environmental testing men came, did air samples, and looked in and under the house.

The results came back as equal to outside. Thank goodness for that. Since that time I have been in other environments for long periods and my lungs never seem to react any differently.

CHAPTER FORTY-FOUR

"A wise person gets known for insight; gracious words add to one's reputation."

Proverbs 16:21 MSG

Persistent described my approach to the clinic and determined described my desire to push an answer from the stalemate around my future. I had kept asking when my job would again be available. Again, the response was, yeah, I want that, but the reality: there was no job waiting. For whatever reason, the promise had dissolved.

Having realized that fact months before, I had wanted an admission from the promise-maker that the job was not there for me anymore. I felt I was due that response. I had not asked for that promise, didn't even expect it. It was made though, and an answer or a rescinding of the offer was owed. That, to me, was the only right way to end the stalemate.

I just wished the finality of the offer would be verbally confirmed. The game was becoming tiresome, this passive-aggressive behavior becoming ever more predictable and boring.

The staff at the clinic had been good to me, always glad to see me when I came by for meds or to say hello. I did not want to take advantage of the situation and thus became especially careful to make appointments. I paid for services at regular price as I went, even though I was told I did not have to pay for what I needed. I felt not doing so would have eventually generated a bad situation. The conversation was the same every time I paid my bill.

"You don't have to pay anything; you know I don't care."

"I know, it's a "me thing." I need to pay."

"OK, but you know I don't care."

Well, I did care. I was not on staff anymore. I paid for my consumption.

During the summer of 2003, Topper had had to have glaucoma surgery. On a particular day in August, I think, I had gone to the clinic to get some medication for Topper's eyes and have his pressure checked. The receptionist set a time right before lunch for my appointment.

Since I was no longer on staff there, I did not feel comfortable in coming in, commandeering a technician and taking care of things myself. I was now a client and paying for the service of expertise and time. Doc acted as if the rules had changed and did not want to help. I asked for the help and finally the pressure was read. I picked up Tops, paid for the meds and headed to the car. I realized it was one of those "damned if you do, damned if you don't" situations. I paid and got in the car to leave. While backing out of the parking lot, Mother spoke.

"Did you notice your name is not on the door anymore?"

"No, I didn't. Is it gone, really?"

I snickered out loud and began shaking my head from side to side, especially after the situation I had just been through. Mom shook her head as well and grinned.

"Yeah, I looked while you were inside with Topper, it is gone."

"Well, you would have thought I would have been told before it was done, or at least afterwards; why not today even?

I was in there for 10 minutes and they all acted rather distant and surly. There was not going to be a single mention of it. What a piece of work."

In all honesty, I was relieved the game was over and did not let it hit the radar screen for long. I just wished it had been dealt with the year before. All it would have taken was a simple repeal of the offer. Life would have settled out sooner for everyone involved. I let it go, having learned a lesson about promises.

I also understood that in my heart I did not care about that job. I had just wanted the offer confirmed or denied and not in a passive-aggressive manner. Head-on is a much better method of dealing with any situation, in my opinion.

My life to point had taught me that a door would open at the right time. The job at this clinic had served its purpose and that purpose was over. At this moment I felt it was more of a respect issue. After one-and-a-half years and the fateful promise, I was owed that answer and in a timely and honest manner. I had to laugh though, remembering the day I was told with all sincerity to not worry, my job would be waiting.

Another of Dad's life lessons without participation on my part came home to roost and drove home one point to me: Make no promise at all or own that you have no intention of doing something. This is much better all the way around.

CHAPTER FORTY-FIVE

> "You gain strength; courage and confidence by every experience in which you really stop to look fear in the face. You must do the thing you think you cannot do."
>
> Eleanor Roosevelt

After we tested the house, Dr. Milstone started me on Azithromycin three times a week, in addition to the Cellcept and the Advair. Breathing came easier for the first time in a year. September 2003 had arrived. Fall came creeping in on air found to be cooler and not so humid: the perfect weather for walking outside and time for me to get after my plan for re-establishing my life once again.

Debbie Swanner is one of my best friends, beginning in our high school days. Life had separated us with time, distance and obligations, but we found our friendship had not faltered over the years. Deb was so important to me during this third time of healing. We would walk every day. Deb is very bright and funny and has always been a talker and a joker, and she would keep me occupied with chatter and laughter; eventually I could climb hills and walk for an hour. I was really going to get there this time. I felt so much stronger.

Dr. Milstone had sent me to respiratory rehab during the summer and I had learned how to eat and breathe correctly, and how to relax in a breathing crisis. All of that helped me keep this cycle of healing moving forward.

Early that fall, Laura had come home and so had my other lifelong friend Nancy Budny. We would all walk together. One day during our walk everyone was steps ahead, laughing and having a vigorous walk. I was not keeping up, a good quarter-mile behind the group. I was getting very tired, breathing labored, my joints were aching, and my muscles were cramping and painful. Noticing I was not with the group Laura turned around saw my state and took me home. That ended that round of healing; back to Vandy once again.

More tests indicated no major change in my lungs, but the disease was progressing. Prednisone again; I went manic, again: same reaction, same temporary suppression of the problem. Before this backslide occured, I had managed to regain some muscle and had gained back weight to 140 pounds, which did not last.

Appointments with Dr. Madan were still scheduled for every three months. By this time in a normal transplant schedule, visits should be once a year if even needed. I would have been re-vaccinated to regain immunity for all those childhood diseases lost when bone marrow is destroyed. Weary was my personal best descriptive for this prolonged post-disease period. Respiratory disease recurrence, not sleeping well because my legs and feet would cramp at night, not understanding how one week I felt great and the next so poorly, was taking its toll on my hope, my patience and my ability to control my attitude about my present state of affairs. I was working so hard to get my body and my life back and I kept falling backwards.

Knowledge helped the first go-'round; I needed more knowledge about this stage of my trek. I wanted and needed every body system checked. There had to be more to this than *just* lung disease. Why was every system bothering me? Why can I not get past all of these nagging additions to my recovery time? I did not like this post-transplant state at all.

Anger and frustration were digging in alongside me, trying to become my permanent companions. A feeling of helplessness fed by the frustration of treatment failure was rearing its head and I was determined that feeling was not going to win. I wanted this stuff gone; I needed my life back. I didn't know who I was anymore. This "stuff in my lungs" was defining what my life would be and I resented the heck out of that fact. I thought I had won my scrape with the reaper. Why was he back at my door? Why can't I get better? Are we missing something?

The seal that had kept all of these bad concepts from forming in my vacuum tube paradise had broken. Air of a new realization was being sucked into my world. The tube was cracking and I was being tossed back into a reality that would have been better left in its state of Pollyannadom. I wanted my ignorance back. I needed my bliss back. I needed my hope back. I was going to find it somehow and soon.

A cardiac workup was scheduled. After the initial stress test, the cardiologist wanted to schedule a cath. Invasive procedures were not something I wanted to undergo. The goal had to be less medical treatment, not more. Would they do a cath just to make sure all bases were covered? All my tests had been relatively normal, similar to what Bishop had found all those years before. I stalled until other tests were done; sound familiar?

Because of the yo-yo life, I was living; I was not in the best of moods. My fuse was shortened because of the stress associated with the lack of positive response by my lung disease. In the past two-and-a-half years I had never been this consistently angry over my lack of progress. The years past found me trudging along, conquering the tiring hills, staying positive and believing life would get better and back to normal. Anger popped in occasionally but it ran away just as soon as I had sensed its presence. The Pollyanna gig, I assume. I trusted my medical team to keep me informed as to my chance in regaining what I had lost. I was depending on them being frank and not holding back. Sometimes they did, sometimes they didn't. But no matter who said what when, I had stayed angry this time around.

Anger was taking a serious toll on my attitude around my doctors. Under normal circumstances I do not like anger to be a part of my life. It takes entirely too much energy to stay in that state of mind. Anger generates a tired soul and a tired body. Bearing a tired soul develops an overall mistrust and an environment for poor decision-making. I was beginning to believe I had misplaced my trust in getting the answers I needed. I felt an overwhelming obsession develop, driving me to know the extent of what was going on with my body and recovery. I felt that my obsession to know left my doctors not caring anymore that I was not getting better. Maybe my quest had exhausted them and they were over it all as well.

Anger lets you think that way. That pattern of thought is one of the main reasons I hate the emotion anger. Anger blunts reality, fogs its edges and robs us of our hope and joy. We are all victims when anger prevails.

All of my life, when I am tired, stressed, frustrated and angry at situations I cry. A feeling of an inability to affect change becomes the driver of the team. I was all of those emotions but I needed them in the moment to give me strength to keep pushing. Giving up and caving in to a lifeless life was not an option. I was still looking for a way out of this mess.

I had had an appointment with Dr. Madan the week before I was to see Dr. Milstone. Angry and probably afraid I would never regain my life; frustration had welled up during that visit with Dr. Madan. I cried. I had never done that before to anyone at Vanderbilt, or at home for that matter. Tears were always an alone thing. I had stressed my family enough with this trial. Tears were my release and they did not have to be shared in their moments of falling.

I was not pleased with myself having collapsed to this level of behavior. Madan recognized my frustration and understandingly gave me a hug and then the oft-repeated motivating phrase about the three-year mark being a golden moment for resolution of a lot of the post-transplant problems. I had to believe in that frame of time.

Regardless, there was a feeling on my part that they also had a role in this particular play in that they failed to manage my final life expectations in a better way. I wanted and expected my life back when I walked out the door of VUMC in October 2001. Many post-transplant patients find a six to 12-month recovery time enough to regain their normal life. Granted, a lot of those folks who have autologous transplants do not have some of the troubles that allogenic transplant people encounter, so they are back in the world much faster. Obviously, my life was not going to fit into one of those molds. I had had an allo and I had hit a wall called lung disease. I was feeling resentment around that loss of rapid recovery.

My life was not a product that could be used and easily replaced with some other choice. I was a human being with an identity composed of many factors and every day I seemed to lose more of me. I was over the hold this disease had on my future. I needed this disease behind me. I wanted my past back.

Mine was not a replaceable life. That was all I knew for sure, wanted and cared about right now. Every time I tried to get going again, something else happened. The end result was a worsening of disease, no matter what I or they did to alter its course. Paul Simon was singing in my head once again and having heard it all of my life I was finally and permanently sick of that refrain and wanted to change the path this journey was taking into the future.

All of the easily grabbed medical, psychological descriptive words that doctors use to describe something driven by emotion or the desire for life lost, like panic attack, anxiety and depression, were coming into play and I resented those assumptions. I was just flat angry and frustrated and tired, and rightfully so. I had fought this lung stuff for two-and-a-half hard years. I was not depressed or having anxiety attacks.

If I was into that phase I would have been sitting at home, I would be fretting and crying constantly, or drinking myself into an alcoholic stupor, giving up and doing absolutely nothing to further my chances at life. I would be in a state of total abandonment of life. I was not near that, I wanted change and I wanted it now.

I resented the implications those labels brought forward. I felt that after what I had lived through to date I deserved a little more compassion than an easy label sticker slapped on my shirt or forehead declaring me not with the program. Labels are too easy and never exact. What was wrong with me was that I needed a positive expectation from somewhere and damned if I was not going to get it one way or another! Another bridge would probably collapse; I had brought my dynamite. It was made up of fear and fright and anger all in one, and would be set off by the need to find some positives to hang onto and go forward.

On my next visit to Vanderbilt, I continued my search for answers. My vascular tree was tested because I had so much leg pain at night and when I exercised. I had just come from the vascular center to keep my next appointment with Dr. Milstone.

Tears were filling my eyes, and as usual my inner conversation began to talk myself down from the moment, trying to make those wet spots go away. I was still incredibly short of breath, and rather gray in color. I had scared the vascular guy while I was on the treadmill. I timidly laughed as I told Milstone I had had a very difficult time during the test.

Already tired of the game, hurt in my spirit, frustrated and angry, I was fighting the urge to break with every ounce of energy I had left. Emotion was about to get my goat and I was powerless to stop the moment from flowing over into the next. I had lost any ability to respond with any level of control.

Milstone sat back in his chair and looked at me with one of those looks like I was crazy.

"Why did you have that done?"

He barked at me. He seemed incredulous.

Here I was, desperately seeking answers as to why I kept living on the teeter-totter of better/worse and then here is Milstone's unsolicited reaction to my search. I felt my need for answers and any tests I had done was no sweat off his nose. His response led me to the knowledge that this meeting was only going to deteriorate into a confrontation. He had challenged my inner search for answers and his reaction set me once again on the defensive.

"Because, my legs are killing me when I try to exercise and vascular disease runs in the family. My legs cramp at night, my joints hurt, I ache all over and I just wanted to make sure my legs were OK."

Granted, he did not know that over the years I had been kicked by horses three times, fallen on once, had a vasculitis the year before, I had had phlebitis in my right leg from my groin to my ankle two years before and had had a non-healing lesion on my lower leg from a biopsy and varicose veins. I felt, and Madan agreed, that I had reason to find out if only for peace of mind over a valid issue. My anger was not abating very much with the response.

"Well, maybe its panic attacks."

That did it! Milstone seemed to me to be patronizing and condescending in the same breath, really pushing the buttons, so to speak. He was now insinuating my health problem was all in my head at this stage and I needed to get over it. I glared, shaking inside so badly I could have erupted like Mr. Creosote, who ate too much in Monty Python's movie *The Meaning of Life*. I have friends that have panic attacks; they have described them to me and, trust me, I have never had one of those types of attacks. I would own it if I did.

"You pick up the phone and you call Deb, you will see I am not having panic attacks. We walk together every day and she knows full well I do not have panic attacks!"

In that moment, his immediate reaction was all that mattered. Milstone kind of backed off, sitting deeper into his chair. That attitude focused my anger to a cone, intensifying it like a laser beam. I verbally lit into him, looking him dead in his eyes.

"You do not know me well enough to assume that pose. This is not a panic attack. I have never had a panic attack in my life and why would I start now? You have no clue as to who I am, what I had been through, or how I have handled it. I think you are a little out of line here!"

I was so angry I probably could have put my fist through the wall. I believe I said that, and that is so "not me." There has only been one other instance in my life where I blew up at another human being. I have always gotten loud over politics, or religion or other topics of conviction. I have never bothered or been pushed to release that much energy at another person over my life's moments. I had never let anyone or anything have that much control over my emotions before.

Our parents raised us to control our emotions but I felt justified this time in letting them control me. It must have been the right thing for me at that moment because the pop-off valve released the pressure and I relaxed all over. I felt that peace I was searching for once more in my soul.

Milstone sat quietly then, looking me in the eye, saying nothing, a stern, impassionate look on his face, a slightly sulking look seeming to block out my response. I came again with the question I had tried so hard to get answered for over a year.

"I want to know why I can't stay well. I am just plain old tired of this game and I am angry! I am over this cycle of getting better and getting worse."

My anger had freed me and backed him into a "medical" corner I could get no one else to enter and loudly and finally I got a reaction:

"Janet, you have chronic lung disease. This is as good as it gets! Now do you see why nobody would tell you that for a year?" I had noticed he had raised his voice that time. I must have pushed his buttons.

Frankly no, I didn't understand why no one would own that result for a year when I had been dealing with it for two years. Why wouldn't they let me in on all the consequences at the beginning of the day? I know they hoped they could stop it, but that wasn't happening, so why not get it out and discussed. I had kept hoping that their lack of finality meant I had a chance of it getting better or going away. It didn't happen. I sat straighter in my chair and breathed out a sigh of conquest. I found what I had gone in search of, hard as it was to get it and hear.

"Thank you. You do not know how long I have been waiting for someone to tell me that and mean it. I can live with that position now and move on."

All I had ever wanted was the truth of what I had, how it was going to play out and a plan for what I could expect. That was all I had ever really been looking for with this search. I needed knowledge.

I knew there was a hint of disgust in my voice. I was sad that it had taken me falling into a whirlpool for someone to throw me the life vest with my new disease's name written all over it. I gathered my stuff and stood up to leave. I was looking for the smoke that always accompanied the bridge collapse.

My new focus was to learn to live within my new parameters, none of which had improved with time. I still had all the joint aches, the cramps; the sleep issues the rapid heart rate the inability to gain weight and difficulty breathing. This was my life now, and it was time my doctors had only a minor part in my life if things were not going to get any better. I just didn't want them to get a whole lot worse. For that goal I still needed my doctors.

Milstone wanted to see me again in three months. I made the appointment and left his office not so sure I would keep it. I left his office heavily laden with sadness and feeling a cold breeze through the huge tear we had created in the fabric of our already threadbare and dysfunctional doctor-patient relationship. I wished it was different. I wished I could see it differently. I was still so mad. Would it ever go away? Would I really be ready and able to move past this moment? I could only pray for something positive or the strength to resolve this anger at my disease state and to learn to move on with my life. I had to believe I was capable of doing that "thing" my fear and anger demanded of me in that moment.

After discussing my position with the cardiologist, I cancelled any further cardiac work-up and left. I informed my family of Milstone's apparent position and they were appalled and offended at his suggestion. Mary just shook her head and stated that I had never had a panic attack and this wasn't one either.

Becky said, "Forget it, Jan."

I knew I was angry about his labeling me so easily and decided to let it go as nothing would be gained by holding on to that moment. The moment had come full circle and was gone. If my family; who has seen me through all sorts of life issues, tells me it is bunk, I trust my own heart and I believe them. It did not make me any less sad that the confrontation had occurred but another dragon was slain, leaving its sulfuric smoking breath hanging around the periphery.

By March 2004, I was again trying to go off the drugs. I was hoping, as Dr. Madan had said, that with time these problems would dissipate. I managed to get through to July and cried "Uncle." I could not breathe. So, back on Cellcept, Advair and Azithromycin and I expect this to be my final state of health. I will not go back on prednisone. That decision is my choice and I have made that choice. A palliative treatment that leaves my life in a mess with a whole new set of medical problems is not how I want to live my life.

My life is now about moving past and through the moment on through to the other side of disease. I am volunteering in a different clinic, trying to regain what not practicing for three years had made me lose. I can manage a couple of half-days and am trying to add more. I plan to start work in January 2005, barring some new problem. I want my life back at whatever level I can have it back. I will succeed in achieving some level of my life, knowing it will not be what it was before January 2000. I have plans for this life God spared. I owe it to Him, to my sister Laura, my family, my friends and to all of my doctors and nurses to get back in the mix for however long my fabric will hold together.

CHAPTER FORTY-SIX

"Get ready; I am going to 'Tub thump,' or lessons I think I've learned."

What a ride! Spare me another, once was enough. Ignorance ran rampant, emotion was dominant, God's wisdom managed to sneak in, and a resultant peace has remained amid the chaos on the other side of disease. I know it is not for me to decide whether you find my lessons credible in your life. This was my journey and they were the lessons I needed to learn to survive or succumb. Take them for what they are, simple journey lessons. Use them if you deem them appropriate. If you find they do not apply, let them go.

These words on paper were my exorcism. I make no apologies for my method or for my conclusions. Much needed to be learned and the time to learn and change accordingly was limited. There was a war to live through, an ordeal that seemed insurmountable and was inescapable. It demanded my absolute presence.

The other side of AMM has left me with yet another mountain to traverse. As with most journeys, I am sure the following lessons will be altered, forgotten or more appreciated with time to look back and re-consider the chosen paths. Especially as I travel through this lung problem I have developed. So, here we go.

Why did I not cave to the poor me category when I was diagnosed with AMM? Why did I almost immediately choose my emboldened soul over the easily obtained desperate soul? My friends ask me this, and the honest answer is I don't know.

On one level, I am sure I responded that way because my family became the rock I could hold to through the passage. God gave me grace to face the trial. My veterinary education gave medical insight for making choices and I was given the blessings of strong friendships and a wonderful medical team.

It seems to me when life's worst fear is recognized, one of two roads is available for travel: one may opt for devastation and resignation or action and resolve to fight, or both at different moments in a disease journey.

Dwelling on the unanswerable question "Why me?" or blaming God for "giving this disease to you" only creates an environment of hopelessness. Precious time is wasted on a question with no answer except, "it is" or "because" or, as an acquaintance once said, "Why not me?" And in my mind God does not "give disease" to anyone, period. Just move quickly through the gravity of this wasted effort and try to live in the day the Lord has made, not in the possibility of future days. Make decisions based on fact, not fear, then fight.

Early on I recognized and appreciated the blessing that this disease was ravaging my body, not my soul. By accepting this fact, I was more able to divorce myself from the emotional attachment we all feel for our shell. This step allowed me to deal with the truths around my plight of transplant.

Recognizing that "I" was safe regardless of the outcome made my passage easier. This lesson still has value to me as I live with my new disease. Know; it is still difficult to accept that I traded one disease for another.

Fear of what your future or lack of one may bring leaves undertones in every moment. This oppressive specter's presence makes it imperative that the person who is sick or dying knows they continue on as an integral part of this world, especially while isolated from their daily life. Isolation perpetuates the fear of having no future.

In isolation it is too easy to give up and give in to fear when the process gets difficult. Know; it does get extremely difficult, and the person who is sick will become lost in a daily struggle to survive. Keeping their mind and soul turned toward the positive and not the trial of the day or the possibility of failure should be the daily goal.

Illness drains a body of all reserve, physical and emotional. All energies are inwardly driven toward survival. Not much energy is left to reassure others of our state.

A patient's family can help by learning to rely on the family unit and the medical staff, not the patient for their personal reassurances of success. The patient has enough to do keeping his or her own mind focused on the trial. I was grateful my family had each other and a good rapport with the doctors, staff and a good base in first-hand medical knowledge.

Life is easier if the support of a patient's dignity and worth becomes a daily mindset from those around them; a priceless and selfless act by friends and family. Losing one's independence to a disease is frustrating, isolating and at times dehumanizing. Patients turn over every aspect of themselves to those who care for them.

Dignity must then be preserved through little acts of giving privacy and showing concern for the feelings of dependence that come with being in the hospital for so long. My world was entirely enclosed within the four walls of 11023 and the underground chamber known as radiology.

You get tired some days, and don't care anymore; you just want it over one way or another. You are poked and prodded daily. You suffer bad or expected reactions to therapy in public as people are present all hours of the day and night. There is no privacy; even your bath is interrupted if the schedule calls for the interruption. You are a body with no space of your own to live in. You are another brick in the wall of the ward.

My only exposure to the world was my window, nurses, doctors, family and, if tolerable, a look at the evening news. I could not read, write, had little energy to converse on the phone and slept most of the time away. Caretakers need to try to give us a world of our own while enmeshed in theirs. We just want space to finish our journey to the other side of disease.

Once we have reached our destination we are given much in that a new contract with a second chance at life has been signed. Patients must demand of themselves the expectation of success and life.

We have become survivors. We managed to wake up one morning and recognize a change in the fabric of our life force had occurred. We have an intimate understanding of the tenuous nature of life.

We know not to begrudge the moment we are living but to trust ourselves to let each precious moment develop into the next. We know our donor gave us the greatest gift on earth. The contract signed with them makes our survival directly and forever linked to the grace of their gift. We know we can never repay that selflessness. We know repayment is not expected but...

We, as receivers of their gift, are forever obligated to do our best to honor our chances in a second life. Our donor's sacrifice deserves the response with another, ours. Thanks to their gift, we have a renewed life; full of a hope and a promise of new bounty that must be shared with others. This mission to share our experience of hope is our sacrifice to that newly regained life. Our knowledge of possibility is now our gift to share.

And share we must. The sphere of sharing may be as small as our family or potentially as large as the world. The size of influence is irrelevant; just share the gift of hope. Share moments of opportunity. Gifts received as a survivor of the grim reaper's attack are screaming to be discovered, explored, seen and shared. Do this with joy and thanks.

I feel survivors cannot become selfish with their life once it is reestablished. We must live for our families, our medical teams and for those who did not survive their journey to the other side of disease. We are now beacons of what can be. Whatever task the new road brings conquer the challenge and be grateful it is offered.

My inner strength and resolve to survive was discovered deep in my being, and eventually I will find a way to share that resolve with others. There were setbacks. But my life goal is to persevere. My path will show itself. I can exclaim that I am a survivor just like Carol said I would be those few short years ago. The inner strength and will to survive that Carol had seen in me is grounded firmly in my faith in God.

God's grace has cared for me all of my life. From the beginning of it, no matter how determined I was to run my life in a ditch, His grace kept me from unknown travails, kept me ignorant of facts I did not need to know, and carried me through difficult moments in my life. I will always acknowledge God as the source of that grace and strength. If there was ever doubt, I now know that prayer, lifted up by thousands, or even one, makes a difference.

God's gift to all patients is our team of medical professionals. No patient arrives at the final destination of greater wellness without unspoken sacrifices from the people who treat our bodies. On the course of this journey to new life, we as patients are focused on the future and tend to forget that the purveyors of that future, the medical staff, are human.

They deserve respect, not a pedestal. They are not perfect. They have cares, concerns, biases, stressors, families, personalities and personal struggles and self-doubt as anyone else in this life. They have good days and bad, like anyone else.

Appreciate their medical abilities in the reference that they are human. Recognizing them as one of us, we need to honor sacrifices they make daily in their lives to care for the lives of others.

People around a transplant patient should expect to be exposed to a human who is emotionally barren and raw. The slightest change will upend us as if a whirlwind screamed through our lives. Daily, patients deal with incredible odds against survival. Daily the need is there for a hint of a successful outcome.

I learned that each member of a transplant family will bear the stress and uncertainty of the time in ways others cannot understand. Outside the circle, people may feel behaviors are unnecessary or irrational or stupid or selfish. We do not owe an explanation.

Patients understand the stress their illness has brought to bear. We never stop worrying about the effect our illness is having on our family. We dwell at times on the effect of the disease on their future and the life we had before its irreparable decline. We are not selfish in our need to be reassured around this moment in our life journey. Honesty, understanding and a clear vision of at least the next day are mandatory for rest and healing.

Defaulting to truth is always the easiest answer in this life of uncertainty, in any given situation, before, during or after. A patient's truth is defined by living in our moments. Our moments are defined by the feeding of our senses and their expression through our emotions.

As patients, we will travel some weird paths before our journey is over, we will show sides of ourselves with raging abandon; at least I did. Most of my hills and valleys came after the transplant was over. My transplant time developed a deeper sense of my spiritual core. Post-transplant really tested my resolve and understanding of the lessons I felt I was to learn.

Recognize that a change in mental state is usually a clear sign of one struggling to reach the next level of healing, of learning how to let go of our old life, or of accepting the final state of health as a result of transplant. Those rollercoaster rides have hills called anger, sadness, happiness, depression, panic, fear, thankfulness, joy, love, peace and acceptance. So let us go there without condemnation.

Traveling through the stages of disease has nothing to do with anyone or anything but the transplant recipient. Emotions are hard to check during this time, so much is happening at once and so much is at stake. Let the emotion out, do not be ashamed of your feelings; let those emotions move through your consciousness, learn from them and then move on.

People around patients need to let those phases pass without taking them personally or assuming the behavior is permanent. Just because a patient's emotional reaction to others or to situations is not what it was before does not mean permanent change in character. Let the moment pass. Leave us to our devices as long as they are not destructive behaviors.

Conversely, patients are not granted carte blanche to forget others have feelings; they should be mindful that their caretakers are hurting also. I am just saying some days will be rougher than others and most of the emotion is aimed at the trial, not the people around the moment.

Outsiders, I mean people who are not in the middle of the journey, should not judge a patient, a patient's journey or their family's response by their personal scale or peripheral reaction to the same scenario. They have no point of reference, only inference based on what they think they would do or how they think they would react. Until you have been told you are dying, until you have lived through a near-death life, sorry, what you think about how someone handles their plight is irrelevant.

Do not judge their moments; let those moments move through you and let them go. For once, it is all about the patient; respect that place. We are fighting for our life or accepting our death or something in-between. Do not expect us to have the emotional strength to deal with much more than our own plight. Give us room to recover.

A transplant patient enters this passage with the knowledge that the option for a new lease on this physical life can be ultimately denied. In the moment of one's acceptance of this possibility, I believe there is a requirement from others to allow the ill individual the freedom to die in peace.

In the humble opinion of one who has had to walk down this road with a possible dead end, I believe firmly that there should be no forcing by others of their fears of loss or their desires for heroic acts upon the person who has already suffered a trial they cannot understand nor fully appreciate.

Granted, all the actors are involved in the struggle: the person who is ill and those who love them and aid them. All have a role to play in the drama. Ultimately all the players will suffer the consequences of a bad play and enjoy the fruits of a good one. Plan well ahead for any decision that may need to be made.

Understand that the decision rests with the one dying and not the living. Gladly allow the peace of acceptance to reign. During this time, we should bring our best to the table; leave life's past difficulties and recriminations in the past. Forgive others and leave it in the past. Bring peace and grace to the life that is leaving. The one who is dying is the only one who has the right to decide their ultimate fate. It is their existence. It is their exit. It is their body. It is their soul.

Having defined that position, the caveat lies in the reality that the dying person owes it to themselves and their family to have made life-ending choices before the trial begins. Not having death's circumstance elucidated before entering the hospital is in my opinion just plain irresponsible. Not preparing ourselves legally, financially and spiritually to die is the ultimate in selfish behavior.

Not preparing for that eventuality leaves our loved ones to assume and guess and suffer through unnecessary days of emotional struggle, trying to find a way to read our minds and discover our desires. They only have their frame of reference to make a decision. That is not enough.

Love your family and yourself enough to be prepared to die. Ignoring death won't make the possibility any less, only more tragic if left ignored. Don't wait until the moment is upon you; work through the labyrinth early and mark the path for others to follow. The path is tortuous and painful but what a great gift for those who love you.

I believe that of all influences upon us the mind is the most dominant. Our mind can literally be for us or against us, but we control that position. Our mind, if left to its own devices, can create such untruths as to prevent us from seeing our path. Seek the truth and deal with it.

Unchecked, our mind can be the greatest harbinger of demons, creating them out of shadows of possibilities, not fact. My mind was always running in high gear through out most of my early diagnostic period. Only later on did I learn how to shut down the persistent noise and get the fear out of the way.

The answer I found was to empower my mind to only find the truth and then to find a path to overcome the adversity presented by that truth. Our mind can help us recognize emotions and patterns that define the truth of our journey. We need to realize they exist and make needed changes. The changes can help define the choices we need to make and understand their consequences.

Fear without basis, or misunderstood truth, keeps us from being present for our life. The created fear always seems worse than the reality that comes from the action. Our monsters under the bed and in the closets of our childhood weren't real. Nor are most of the thoughts that travel through our brain during this time of our lives. Trust yourself, believe in what you know to be true in your life and use your mind to your benefit.

Yes, our body has suffered but we can move forward. There will be times when the ordeal becomes a real nuisance. In these moments, dig deeper and gain the strength to take the next step. Always, keep your mind in check and keep thinking forward.

Transplant patients fear chemotherapy and radiation because they change us visibly. These treatments cause both temporary and sometimes permanent change in some tissues. These treatments may predispose one to develop other medical challenges, some deadly or some to be lived with at some level for the rest of life.

A litany of some transplant consequences might be: lost body hair (regenerates and usually with a temporarily different color and /or texture), dry skin (permanent in my case), varying degree of dry eyes (permanent in my case), food tasting only of salt because all of the taste buds die off (again temporary, mine lasted about a year), oral and intestinal lesions (temporary, gone shortly after I finished Methotrexate), cataract formation (mine began about three years after my transplant and should be surgically removable), eventual loss of thyroid gland function (usually within five years of transplant and again medically treatable), lung and heart disease (usually not a good result if occurs, witness myself), and a slight increase in the chance for the development of soft tissue cancers (may or may not be treatable, witness David).

The side effects and results of treatment are the future we accepted by signing the dotted line. The problem comes in the recognition that sometimes we as patients have forgotten all the agenda and the costs of our journey. Realization of one of these consequences is disheartening after such a long fought battle.

Because we forget or temporarily dispel the possibility of these outcomes, I feel that our transplant center teams need to really manage post transplant outcome expectations. Patients embedded in the day-to-day do not focus on the long-term. We may or may not have a long-term. If a patient gets past that stage, the need to really understand what comes with living must be addressed again.

These do not need to be cursory conversations nor platforms for alarmism. Topics with lifelong implications should be revisited in compassionate, understandable doses, Mary Poppins' spoonful of sugar method, if you will. A gentle reminder of our price to pay is all that is needed in the moment.

There were moments while in the hospital in which I did feel that my team was not so available to discuss these topics. They were busy, had many patients to see, patients in more need of them than I at some moments, but still they should have found time for these kinds of conversations during the treatment. If not discussed during the treatment then certainly discuss them as they live out their one hundred days.

Realities take a toll when they start to present themselves on a daily basis, and the pre-transplant conversation is too old in a patient's mind and we are probably too tired and sick going into the treatment for them to have been of much help in the long run.

Doctors should not assume we won't understand the cause and effect we are living. They should not assume we do not want to talk about the future or the lack of one. Doctors have a skill we as patients lack.

Doctors' daily experiences with people in all walks of life and all stages of disease teach them when different levels are in play. Because of this unique position, I think doctors could really participate in this journey by recognizing a transplant patient's steps along the path of healing. They could call or explain the behavior if needed and help the patient find the way to the root of their emotional place, whatever that root is.

Calling behavior is a difficult thing to do but it is a valuable tool that is sometimes ignored amid the din of survival. If necessary, add psychological care to in hospital options for those in need of help finding a path through their maze, or through their sadness, or anger or their as yet unrecognized feelings.

Dr. Milstone, although I am sure not his original intent because of the unexpected encounter with my moment of fulminate anger, had the opportunity to call the stage for me during my last appointment. He was at first an agitator and then a passive filter. He allowed the vocalization of my anger at a situation, not him, flow through him. He sat there, quiet, focused, mostly professional and mostly impassionate.

He let me release all that anger I had ignored for several months. Know; I was not comfortable as it erupted. I despised myself in those moments of anger. As I said before, anger, to me, is the worst emotion around. But, the release of that anger freed me to realize and own that over the years that followed the transplant I had given my own power to my disease state and the doctors who cared for me.

I was ignorant of my reality of living from episode to episode, appointment to appointment, with the fear of not living completely again. My family's fears for my future or lack of one aided the dependence. One very important lesson came to light.

A patient's ability to give up power over their life because of the fear of not living or fear of not being able to find a new life is an easy trap to fall into when facing the "death of the old-in with the new" life issue.

We cling to those who have the ability to carry us across the bridge to health. They become the pied pipers that we follow toward the light at the end of the tunnel. And we, like rats mesmerized by their tune, run and stuff our souls with that presence of hope in our life. Doctors become our earthly assurance that we are still surviving, hope lives in those assurances.

My last appointment with Dr. Milstone created an environment that allowed me to recognize the existence of a cord still attaching me to Vanderbilt in a way that I thought I had moved past. That open and confrontational environment sparked by our dysfunction gave me the strength to sever that cord.

That moment of grace has been the greatest blessing received on the other side of this disease. The anger in our confrontation allowed me to free myself from the chains of being an ill person, the chains of the appointment cycle and the dependence upon being reassured. It allowed me to break that final chain link of fear that was keeping me from putting the death march behind me and heading back into the world with what I had left of the old me. Daddy would have called the realization a 2 x 4 to the head. I recognized it as just that, as I have had much experience with that particular attention-getter.

Patients, always be mindful of that attachment forming. We need the attachment early on; it is the landmark of time passing and that we are still living. The important thing about bonds, though, is that given enough energy (mine was in the form of anger), the inertia of sameness is overcome and we are ready to help cut the attachment and move on to the next level of our healing. Move toward this healing with joy and excitement and move past the disease. Move toward your new life.

This step is mandatory to get your life back into your own hands. Recognize it will be a new life, not the one you had before. Embrace the newness and be thankful for the energy surge you found to get past the dependence.

As Emerson said, "A foolish consistency is the hobgoblin of little minds..." I was foolishly consistent in living as patient. Illness had become my mind's hobgoblin. I had to break the cycle. I did.

Families need to understand that the patient eventually has to regain their status as a contributing person of the world. I had a few setbacks. Each setback caused my family's fears to rise again. They immediately went into their protect Janet mode. I love that they love me.

The truth is that now they need to let me go back into the world and let me take my chances with whatever time I have left in this new life. I know they will never let me off the leash; fine, give me room to run. Let me fail if need be; it won't be the first time I failed. I hope it won't be the last.

As an adult patient I still found the effect of my parents' control on my future immense. As a child you tend to push and fight the control your parents exert over your life. Had I not had my father and mother as role models, I cannot say that I would have fared through this ordeal as well as I did. God blessed me with a wonderful pair of loving, wise, strong parents. The love for their children was greater than any other aspect of this world. Their sacrifices were great and constant. They taught us to survive.

No doubt, I have the greatest bunch of siblings in the world, warts and all. I pray all families could know this kind of love. Their sacrifices were great and immediate, grand displays of the job our parents did in creating a family. I love my siblings more than my own life and would give it for them without thought.

Mary and Don are angels on this earth. They are compassionate, giving, loving people. What a blessing to have them in my family.

I had opportunities and lessons presented to me during my journey from different people for different reasons. I have learned that some people in the greater world grow weary of your health or lack of it. The post-disease relationship will always be altered, and not necessarily for the better. That is a sad and unnecessary result, in my opinion.

I learned how some people can act with compassion but ultimately they are found essentially deceptive in their behaviors and found self-focused. Some people are so self-involved they never give of themselves, except on a cursory level, and have an inability to recognize need in anyone else but themselves.

On the opposite end of that spectrum, I learned that some people are so selfless you wonder how they survive in this world at all. There are people in our lives that will be there come hell or high water. These people are God's gifts to our lives. Take care of these relationships. Cherish them and hold them close. The presence of a true friend is one of the most precious gifts of grace in our lives.

I have every intention to get back to riding horses. I pray my body agrees with me. Maybe one day I will have my big grey Trakener grazing in the pasture. The reality, probably will not.

I have a goal to minimize my need for medical attention. I must learn to live with just enough of that presence.

I have a goal to be able to support myself again without SSA. But, I know that because of my lung issue and my thin, weak body I may never really achieve that goal. I will try.

I have a goal to never forget what I have been through, to never forget the grace that I had been shown and been given, to never forget the lessons learned or of the relationships made and lost, and will always cherish my love for my family and God.

I have learned that one should attack life with gusto and not tolerate it in silence. Learn to push limits, to face adversarial positions head on and to not be afraid to express opinion or test gifts.

Fear of failure is not a dominant factor in my choices anymore. My life question has become, "Why not?" We are responsible for our own failures and our own successes. We each live with our own what-ifs and only ourselves to blame for our lack of "Why did I not try?"

I recognize that my life will have a new timbre from now on. I am much more mindful of my weaknesses, and much more active in trying to contain them and move through them. I have tried to find new talents, and I think I have.

I hope my journey helps someone on a similar path see that life affords us the grace for the challenges we face that seem insurmountable. Learn how to recognize blessings when they present themselves along the path and overcome your hardship. Lessons come in odd packages so don't be afraid to open them and celebrate the gift we receive inside the box.

I wish for all transplant patients, all patients with life-threatening disease, the peace that love can give. I wish grace for them and their families. I wish great skill and knowledge for their doctors and the peace of knowing life goes on.

Know that I feel I found a place that God allowed me to live in through this experience. By my learning to let go of my life and letting God take that life, it allowed me to live my life.

As transplant survivors we need to recognize the gift of life, not remain in the state of flux called disease. My unsolicited advice: go, find new talents, really love those precious souls in your life and try to find a way to use your talents and gifts to give back to others.

The caveat: your future options may take a while before they become apparent. Just know in your soul that they will appear. So be open to new opportunities and when presented with those opportunities, take them and run. Stay optimistic, be compassionate toward others, and give of yourself freely as you pass through the journey and survive.

If, over time, my lung disease worsens and I lose what I have regained, I pray I will be thankful for the grace period given my life after AMM. The other side of disease is a wonderful time to begin again. I want to use it wisely.

EPILOGUE OCTOBER 22, 2004.

Today is overcast; fall is quickly coming in the South. Trees are not yet at peak color and the air is jacket-cool. I have a jacket on today: red and blue corduroy with stars, like our flag.

My three-month visit is due and Madan has ordered a chest CT, blood work and pulmonary function tests. Testing is complete my appointment with Dr. J. is for 2:30. I brought my camera this time. There are several people and places I want a memento of for this book and my memory bank.

I found my nurses, my doctors, the locations and objects inside the hospital who all played a role in my journey. No photo was taken without permission. A few outside shots were in order. Vanderbilt is imposing.

Walking out the front door of the hospital and turning to the left I photographed the brick and concrete sign proclaiming the site. Moving into the turn around area, I found the hospital in my viewfinder. It didn't fit; I had to take two or three shots. I turned left and took shots of the walkway bridges. Amazing and awe-inspiring are the only words that fit this building.

I placed my camera back in its carrier and headed toward the library. My plan included searching for information on family member attendance to the Vanderbilt Dental School of the 1900s. About one-third the distance to the Heard library a voice behind said, "Excuse me; ma'am?"

A few more steps and I recognized I was ma'am. I stopped and turned, "Yes."

There was a young man in police fatigues behind me.

He smiled, "Vanderbilt Police, ma'am."

I started to laugh. "You want to know why I was taking pictures of the hospital, don't you?"

He dropped his head a little, grinned, "Yes ma'am."

I told him my reasons for taking the photos.

He smiled. "You are on public property and you haven't done anything wrong."

"Oh, I know; it's OK, you are just doing your job. The library is this way, isn't it?"

"Oh, yes, ma'am, walk past the Nursing School and on the other side of that big tree you will see the steps. Have a good day." He turned and walked back to his duty site.

"Thanks. You too."

I thought about the Southern-ness of the conversation, and in the directions to the library. Go past the big tree. Yes, ma'am, no, ma'am: polite, respectful, to the point and in a non-threatening manner. I love the South, but the encounter left me feeling a little disconcerted. 9/11 was still here; this time it had affected me in a quite different way.

I am a white, American female in her early 50s, taking photographs of the institution that saved her life. I am suspect. I keep hearing Paul Simon, Proust and Gray.

That encounter aside, my lungs are still not normal but thought not to be deteriorating anymore to point; my blood counts are holding and the DNA is still all Laura, so I think AMM is truly history. I am alive, enjoying the gifts given, and enjoying my family and friends, participating as fully in this life as I find possible. I still wake up daily at sunrise and thank God for his blessings and his grace. I am still letting go and letting God.

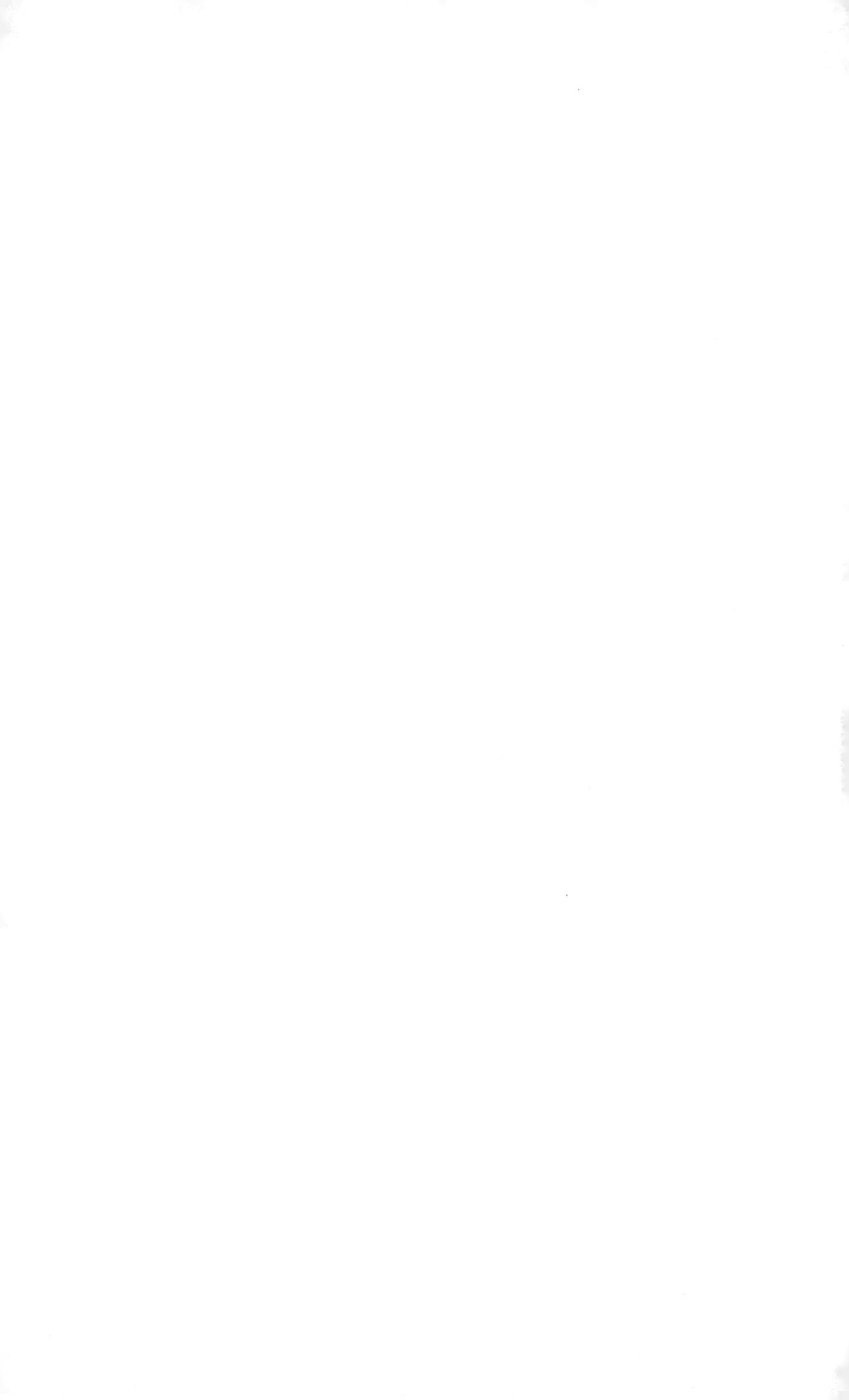